# RADIOLOGY

## for Undergraduates and General Practitioners

# RADIOLOGY

## for Undergraduates and General Practitioners

**Hariqbal Singh** MD DMRD
Professor and Head
Department of Radiology
Shrimati Kashibai Navale Medical College
Pune, Maharashtra, India

*Co-author*

**Dinesh Pardesi** MD
Consultant
Department of Radiology
Shrimati Kashibai Navale Medical College
Pune, Maharashtra, India

JAYPEE

**JAYPEE BROTHERS MEDICAL PUBLISHERS**
*The Health Sciences Publisher*
New Delhi | London

**Jaypee Brothers Medical Publishers (P) Ltd**

**Headquarters**
EMCA House
23/23-B, Ansari Road, Daryaganj
New Delhi 110 002, India
Landline: +91-11-23272143, +91-11-23272703
+91-11-23282021, +91-11-23245672
E-mail: jaypee@jaypeebrothers.com

**Corporate Office**
4838/24, Ansari Road, Daryaganj
New Delhi 110 002, India
Phone: +91-11-43574357
Fax: +91-11-43574314
E-mail: jaypee@jaypeebrothers.com

**Overseas Office**
J.P. Medical Ltd
83 Victoria Street, London
SW1H 0HW (UK)
Phone: +44 20 3170 8910
E-mail: info@jpmedpub.com

**EU GPSR** Authorised Representative
Logos Europe, 9 rue Nicolas Poussin
17000, La Rochelle, France
Phone: +33 (0) 6 67 93 73 78
E-mail: contact@logoseurope.eu

Website: www.jaypeebrothers.com
Website: www.jaypeedigital.com



**Inquiries for bulk sales may be solicited at:** jaypee@jaypeebrothers.com

**Radiology for Undergraduates and General Practitioners**
First Edition: 2012
**Reprint: 2026**
ISBN 978-93-5025-793-7
*Printed at: Samrat Offset Pvt. Ltd.*

**Dedicated to**

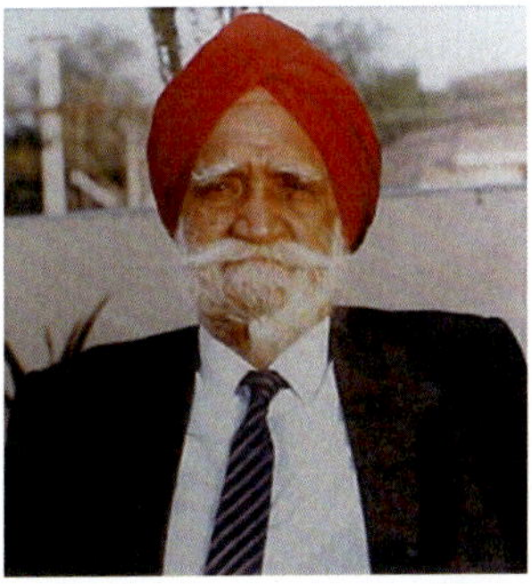

*My dear father Harnam Singh on his 101st birthday*

*Radiology is a Kindergarten*
*of logical rational coherent exploration and balanced learning*
*and not*
*dexterous adroit smugness*
*or learning egotism*
*cultivated by fake self-centeredness and egoism.*

***–Hariqbal Singh***

# Contributors


**Amol Nade** DMRE
Consultant (Radiology)
Shrimati Kashibai Navale Medical College
Narhe, Pune, Maharashtra, India

**Sushil G Kachewar** MD (Radiology)
Associate Professor
Rural Medical College
Loni, Rahata, Ahmednagar
Maharashtra, India

**Abhijit Pawar** DNB (Radiology)
Assistant Professor
Shrimati Kashibai Navale Medical College
Narhe, Pune, Maharashtra, India

**Shailendra Savale** DNB
Consultant (Radiology)
Shrimati Kashibai Navale Medical College
Narhe, Pune, Maharashtra, India

**Parvez Sheik** DMRE
Consultant (Radiology)
Shrimati Kashibai Navale Medical College
Narhe, Pune, Maharashtra, India

# Preface

*Radiology for Undergraduates and General Practitioners* is a comprehensive book meant for MBBS students who have a wide curriculum and many subjects. In radiology, there is no separate examination but forms part of surgery, however, radiology-related questions are asked in medicine, gynecology and obstetrics.

The syllabus in radiology at undergraduate level is extensive and time is short. The book has been structured such that the student is introduced to radiology and at the same time is prepared to do well in the examination without taking too much of his time. Images have been provided to give a better understanding of the subject. The book covers all questions asked in the examination. At the end of the book, syllabus in radiology for undergraduates has been given. It is expected to be covered in 20 lectures of one hour duration each and one clinical postings of two weeks in radiology department, which is most dubious.

The book will be a great asset for the general practitioners who will find his day-to-day imaging solutions in this.

**Hariqbal Singh**
**Dinesh Pardesi**

# Acknowledgments

We thank Professor MN Navale, Founder President, Sinhgad Technical Education Society, and Dr Arvind V Bhore, Dean, Shrimati Kashibai Navale Medical College, Narhe, Pune, Maharashtra, India, for their kind acquiescence in this endeavor.

We profusely extend our gratefulness to the consultants Anand Kamat, Prashant Naik, Santosh Konde, Amol Sasane, Rahul Ranjan, Rajlaxmi Sharma, Manisha Hadgaonkar, Vikas Ojha, Varsha Rangankar, Aditi Dongre, Yasmeen Khan, Roshan Lodha and Sumeet Patrikar, for their genuine help in building up this educational entity.

Our gratitude to Anna Bansode and Sachin Babar for their clerical help.

We are thankful and grateful to God Almighty and mankind who have allowed us to have this wonderful experience.

# Contents

# 1 CHAPTER

# Musculoskeletal System

**Chapter Outline**



## PATTERNS OF FRACTURE

A fracture is a break in the continuity of a bone. It is important to assess the pattern of fracture as they can indicate the nature of causative violence.

The patterns of fracture are:

1. Incomplete fracture involves only one cortical surface of the bone (Fig. 1.1A).

2. Complete fracture involve both the cortices with displaced or undisplaced fracture fragments (Fig. 1.1B).
3. Linear fracture could be transverse, oblique or spiral fracture. Transverse fracture is a fracture which forms an angle less than 30° with the horizontal line (Fig. 1C). In oblique or spiral fractures, the angle is equal to or more than 30° with the horizontal line (Figs 1.2A and B),
4. Comminuted fracture (Fig. 1.2C) is characterized by three or more fracture fragments.
5. Segmental fracture is one in which the bone breaks into segments at two or more levels, there may be longitudinal split or comminuted fracture (Fig. 1.3A).
6. Impacted fracture occurs when distal fragment of bone is driven into the proximal fragment.
7. Avulsion fracture involves pulling loose of bony insertion by a muscle or ligament (Fig. 1.3B).
8. Hairline fracture is an undisplaced fracture with a fine fracture line (Fig. 1.3C).
9. Occult fracture is suspected clinically but is not visualized on initial radiographic examination.

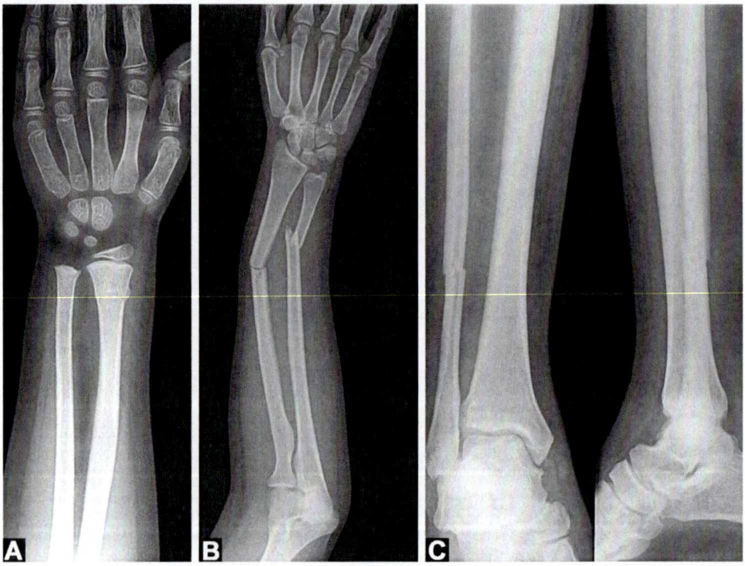


**Figs 1.1A to C:** X-rays show: (A) Incomplete fracture; (B) Complete fracture; (C) Linear transverse fracture

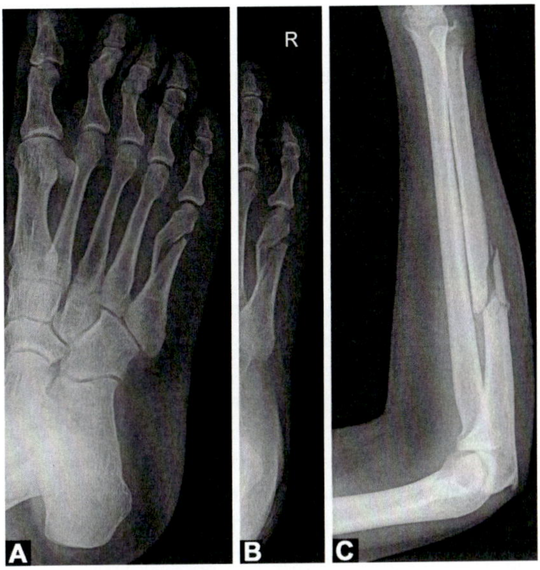


**Figs 1.2A to C:** X-rays show: (A and B) Linear spiral oblique fracture; (C) Comminuted fracture

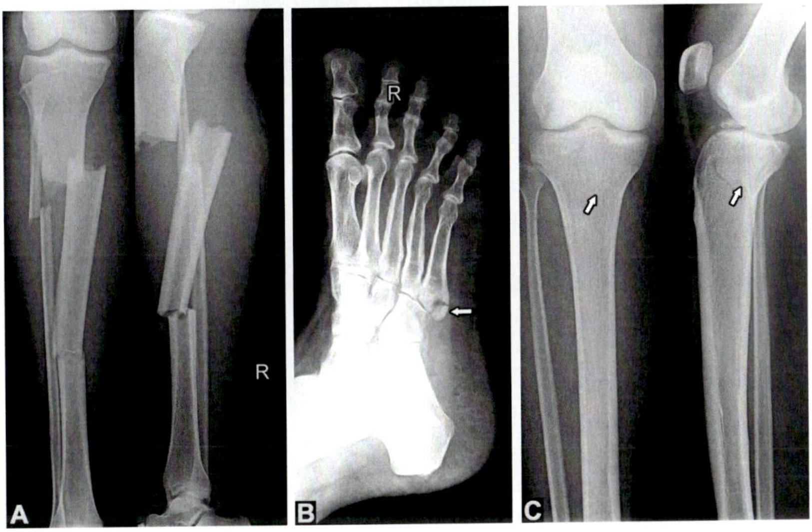


**Figs 1.3 A to C:** X-rays show: (A) Segmental fracture; (B) Avulsion fracture (arrow); (C) Hairline fracture (arrow)

## HEALING OF FRACTURE

The pathological process of healing of a fractured bone occurs in the following stages.

1. Hematoma formation.
2. Subperiosteal and endosteal cellular proliferation.
3. Callus formation.
4. Consolidation.
5. Remodeling.

Initially, there is hematoma formation which is limited by stripped periosteum. In case of torn periosteum, the hematoma is limited by the muscles, fascia and skin. This is followed by stage of cellular proliferation in the subperiosteum and endosteum in the fractured fragments, which gradually develop towards each other, with the absorption of blood clot. The cellular tissue matures to form osteoblasts, which lays down an intercellular matrix, the matrix is then impregnated with calcium and this is callus formation and this is the first radiological sign that indicates healing of fracture. The callus gradually transforms into more mature bone with a lamellar structure in the form of periosteal reaction, leading to union or consolidation of the fracture. After this, there is remodeling stage with gradual strengthening of the bone along the lines of stress.

Factors which influence healing process are:

a. Efficacy of immobilization
b. Interposition of soft tissue
c. Alignment of fracture fragments vascular and neural integrity
d. Local and systemic disease
e. Age of the patient.

Radiological criteria of union are demonstration of visible callus, bridging of the fracture fragments (Fig. 1.4) and blending them with continuity of bony trabeculae across the fracture.

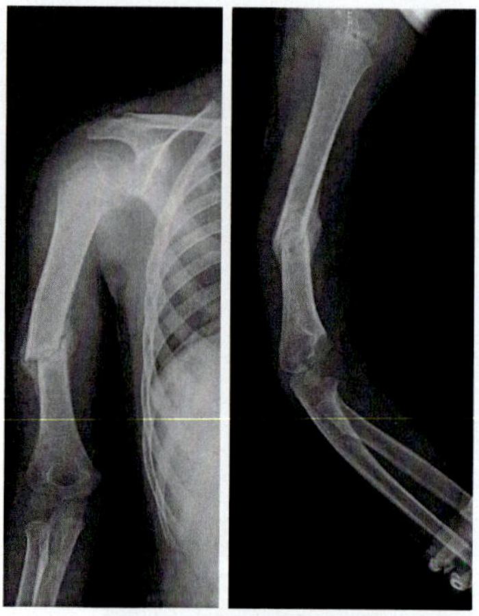

**Fig. 1.4:** X-ray shows fracture of midshaft humerus with callus formation and bridging of the fractured fragments

## FALL ON OUTSTRETCHED HAND

Fall on outstretched hand can lead to injuries at the level of arm, elbow, forearm and wrist.

1. Common injuries at various levels are:
   a. Arm
      i. Fracture proximal humerus
      ii. Oblique/spiral fracture of shaft of humerus
   b. Elbow
      i. Supracondylar fracture of humerus takes place due to mechanism hyperextention at elbow with vertical stress. It is a transverse fracture line and the distal fragment posteriorly displaced/tilted (Fig. 1.5)
      ii. Dislocation of elbow joint
      iii. Radius head fracture
      iv. Fracture of capitellum

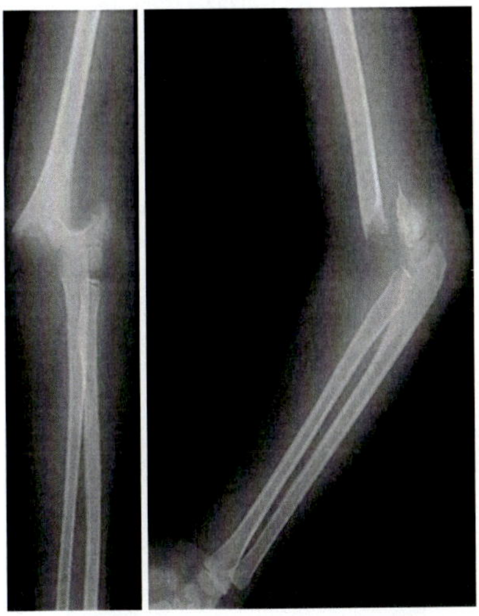

**Fig. 1.5:** Supracondylar fracture

   c. Forearm
      i. Colle's fracture
      ii. Monteggia fracture dislocation
      iii. Galeazzi fracture mechanism is fall on outstretched hand with elbow flexed radial shaft fracture with subluxation/dislocation of distal radioulnar joint (Fig. 1.6)

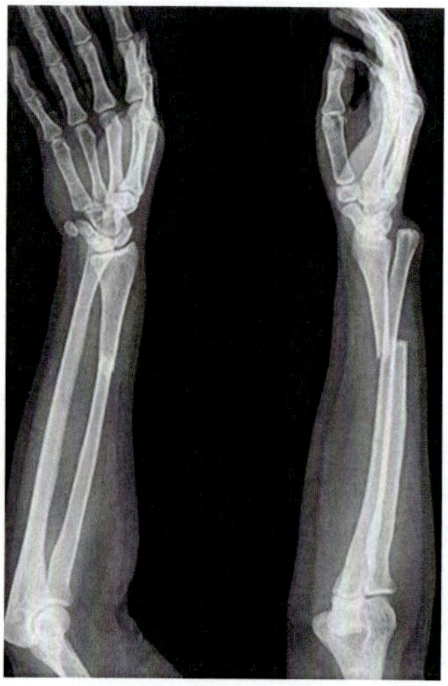

Fig. 1.6: Galeazzi fracture

d. Wrist
   i. Scaphoid fracture (Fig. 1.7)
   ii. Dorsal chip radius fracture
   iii. Lunate and other carpal bone fractures

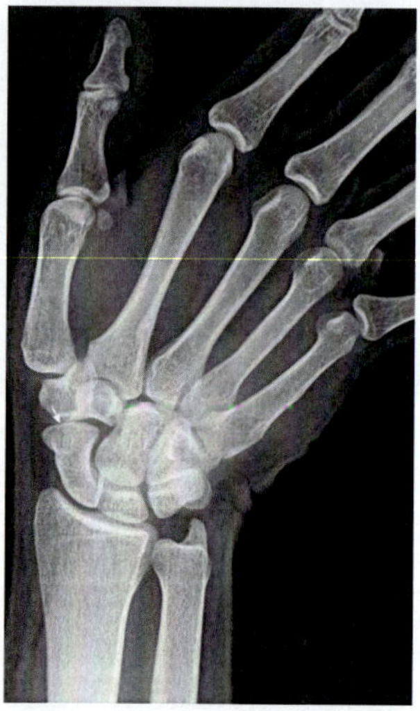

Fig.1.7 Scaphoid fracture

Common fractures at the distal end of forearm or radius following a fall on outstretched hand are:

1. Smith's fracture is reverse Colle's fracture; the mechanism involved is hyperflexion with fall on back of hand. It is nonarticular distal radial fracture with ventral displacement of fragment (Figs 1.8A and B).

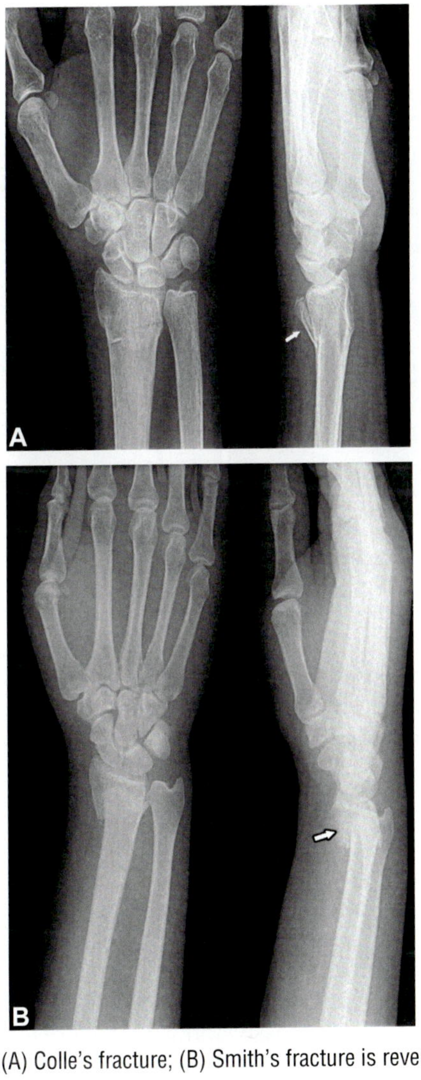

**Figs 1.8A and B:** (A) Colle's fracture; (B) Smith's fracture is reverse Colle's fracture

2. Barton's fracture is intra-articular oblique fracture of ventral or dorsal lip of distal radius (Fig. 1.9A).
3. Chauffeur's fracture also known as Hutchinson, backfire or lorry driver fracture. The mechanism involved is direct trauma to radial side of wrist sustained from recoil of crank; vintage vehicles were started with a crank resulting in acute dorsiflexion and abduction of hand. This resulted in distal radial styloid process fracture of triangular appearance (Fig. 1.9B).

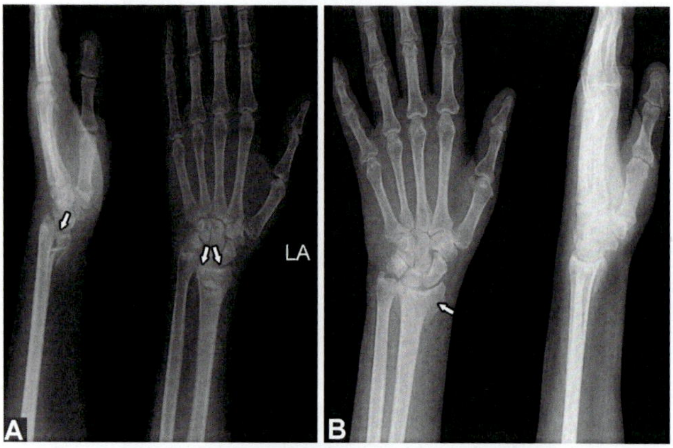


**Figs 1.9A and B:** (A) Barton's fracture; (B) Chauffeur's fracture is also known as Hutchinson, backfire or lorry driver fracture

## RICKETS

It is a metabolic disease of childhood in which the osteoid, the organic matrix of bone, fails to mineralize due to interference with calcification mechanism. It manifest between six months to three years of age.

### Etiology

1. Vitamin D deficiency due to reduced dietary intake, pigmented skin or reduced exposure to sunlight.
2. Malabsorption due to celiac disease, biliary atresia, hepatic osteodystrophy and small intestine bypass surgery.
3. Anticonvulsant therapy.

The characteristic changes are seen in the growth plates prior to closure. Zone of maturation is grossly abnormal. There is overall diminished quantity of calcified osteoid and increase in uncalcified osteoid.

X-rays long bones show widening of the growth plate; this is the earliest specific radiological change. The metaphyseal margins are irregular due to fraying and disorganization of the spongy bone. This results in widening and cupping of the metaphysis (Fig. 1.10). CT scan is generally not required, however will show the changes better as compared to X-ray (Figs 1.11A to D). Epiphysis is osteopenic and there is delayed appearance of the ossification center.

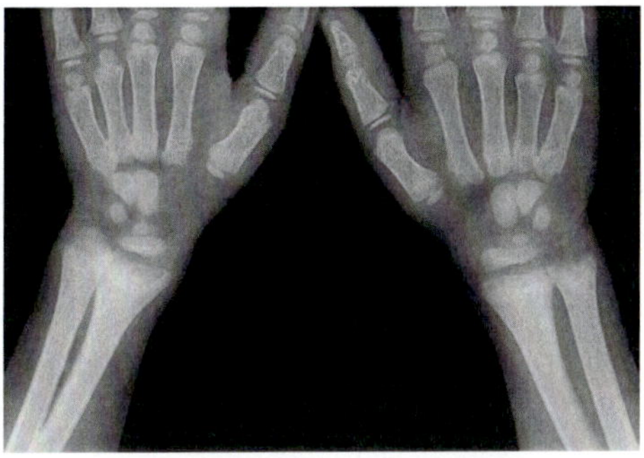

**Fig. 1.10:** X-rays both wrists show widening of the growth plate, the metaphyseal margins are irregular and widened resulting in cupping of the metaphysis

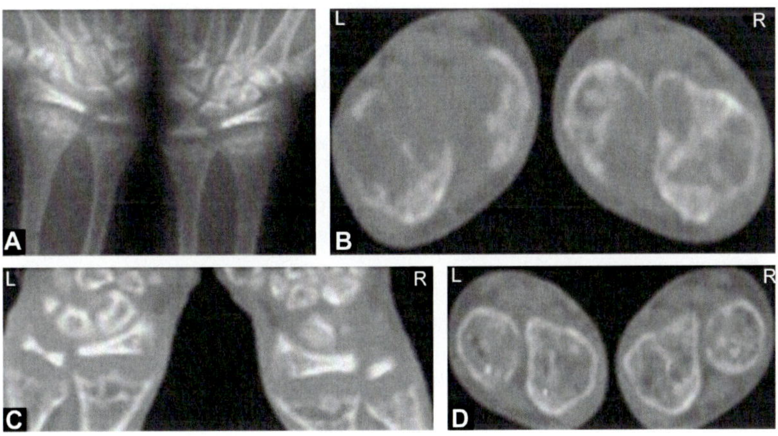


**Figs 1.11A to D:** (A) X-ray of both wrists and hands shows osteomalacia with widening of growth plate, splaying and cupping of distal metaphysis of radius and ulna with irregular metaphyseal margins; (B to D) CT axial and coronal reconstructed images confirm the X-ray findings of defective mineralization of osteoid tissue in cortical and cancellous bone. These are features of rickets

Skeletal deformities include broadened forehead, frontal and parietal bossing.

Pigeon chest is seen due to prominent sternum, narrow chest, ricket rosary (enlargement of costochondral junction) and Harrison's sulci due to diaphragmatic pull on soft ribs. There is exaggerated curvature of spine, trefoil shaped pelvis, coxa vara, genu valgum and bowed tibia.

Treatment is by oral vitamin D—6 lakh IU and same dose is given again after 3 to 4 weeks if no healing sign is seen on X-ray at the metaphyseal end. Followed by a maintenance dose of 4000 IU oral vitamin D if the child is responsive.

## OSTEOPOROSIS AND OSTEOMALACIA

Osteoporosis is a metabolic disorder characterized by decreased mass per unit volume of a normally mineralized bone due to loss of bone proteins. Where as Osteomalacia is a metabolic disorder characterized by failure of mineralization and excess of the unmineralized osteoid due to a derangement in calcification (Table 1.1). It is an adult equivalent of rickets.

### Causes

1. Primary osteoporosis (senile or postmenopausal).
2. Immobilization due to fracture (Fig. 1.12) prolonged bed rest or paralysis.
3. Endocrine-thyrotoxicosis, hypogonadism, hyperprolactinemia, diabetes mellitus, hyperparathyroidism, glucocorticoid excess.
4. Prolonged use of drugs like heparin, ethanol.
5. Nutritional diet-chronic alcoholism.
6. Chronic illness like rheumatoid arthritis, cirrhosis, renal tubular acidosis.
7. Neoplasm—multiple myeloma, leukemia, lymphoma, mastocytosis.
8. Genetic abnormalities—homocystinuria, Ehler-Danlos syndrome, osteogenesis imperfecta.

**Table 1.1** Difference between osteoporosis and osteomalacia

| Osteoporosis | Osteomalacia |
|---|---|
| *Etiology* | *Etiology* |
| i Primary osteoporosis—senile or postmenopausal | i Lack of dietary intake of vitamin D |
| ii Immobilization due to prolonged bed rest or paralysis | ii Decreased absorption of vitamin D—malabsorption syndrome, partial gastrectomy |

*Contd...*

*Contd...*

| **Osteoporosis** | **Osteomalacia** |
|---|---|
| iii Endocrine—glucocorticoid excess, thyrotoxicosis, hypogonadism, hyperprolactinemia, diabetes mellitus, hyperparathyroidism<br>iv Diet—chronic alcoholism, anorexia nervosa<br>v Prolonged use of drugs like heparin, ethanol<br>vi Chronic illness like rheumatoid arthritis, cirrhosis, renal tubular acidosis<br>vii Neoplasm—multiple myeloma, leukemia, lymphoma, mastocytosis<br>viii Genetic abnormalities—homocystinuria, Ehler-Danlos syndrome, osteogenesis imperfecta, Marfans syndrome<br>ix Hepatic disease | iii Deficiency of vitamin D metabolism—chronic renal tubular disease, anticonvulsant therapy<br>iv Decreased deposition of calcium in the bone due to drugs like diphosphonates |
| *Imaging* | *Imaging* |
| Ground glass appearance due to generalized rarefaction | Generalized osteopenia |
| Loss of vertebral body height due to symmetric transverse compression | Loss of transverse trabeculae |
| No looser's zones | Looser's zones at axillary margin of scapula, ramus of pubis or ischium, femur neck, ribs, protrusio acetabuli and triradiate pelvis |
| Pathological fractures at wrist, hip | Pathological fractures |
| Anterior wedge compression and codfish vertebrae | Codfish vertebral bodies due to biconcave vertebral bodies |
| *Treatment* | *Treatment* |
| Calcitonin, sodium fluoride, diaphosphonates, estrogen replacement | Calcium, vitamin D, high protein diet |

### Fractures Due to Osteoporosis

a. At the sites of labile trabecular bone

   Vertebrae:

   i. Anterior wedge compression fracture
   ii. Biconcave vertebral bodies (codfish)

   Wrist-Colle's fracture

b. At the sites of cortical and trabecular bone—Hip-fracture neck femur
c. Fractures of long bone.

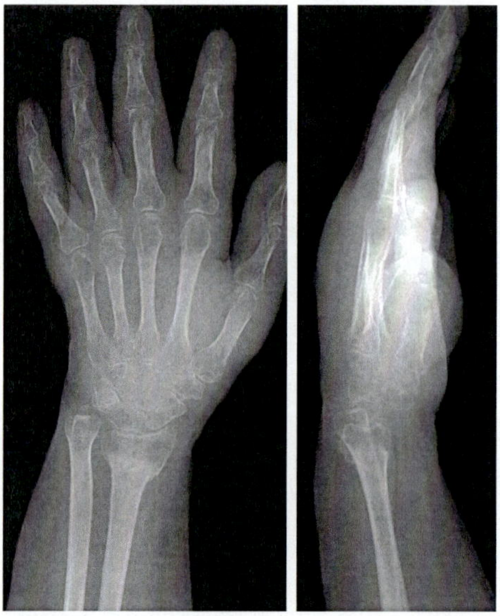

Fig. 1.12: X-ray hand in a post-traumatic patient reveals generalized osteoporosis of wrist and hand bones

## COLLE'S FRACTURE

Colle's fracture is the fracture of lower end of the radius at 2.5 cm above the carpal extremity of radius with fracture dislocation of the inferior radi-oulnar joint. It is characterized by dorsal displacement, dorsal tilt, lateral displacement, lateral tilt, impaction and supination of the distal fragment or fragments (Fig. 1.13).

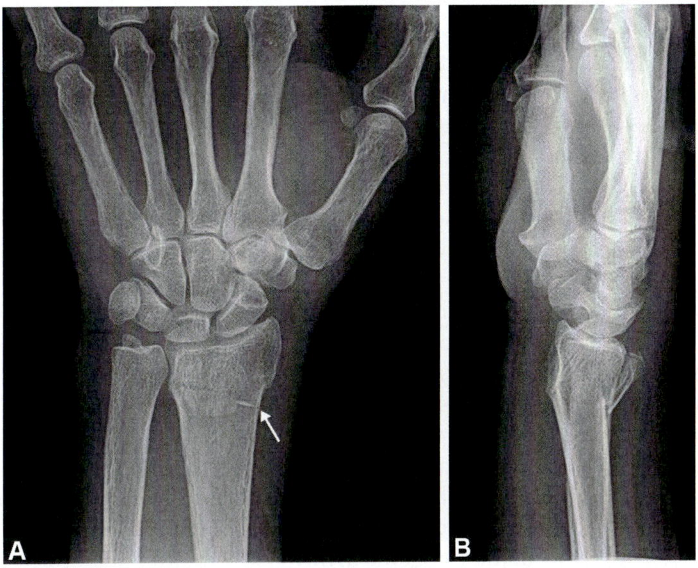


**Fig. 1.13:** Colle's fracture

## Complications of Colle's Fracture

### *Early Complications*

a. Post reduction swelling
b. Injury to proximal segment of bone
c. Median or ulnar nerve damage
d. Compartment syndrome.

### Late Complications

a. Malunion
b. Rupture of the extensor pollicis longus
c. Sudeck's osteodystrophy
d. Frozen shoulder
e. Carpel tunnel syndrome
f. Nonunion.

## ACUTE OSTEOMYELITIS

Osteomyelitis is infection of cortical bone and its marrow space. Osteomyelitis can be caused by bacteria, viruses, mycobacteria or *Treponemas*. Pyogenic osteomyelitis is the most common. It is classified into three forms: acute, subacute and chronic.

Acute osteomyelitis is generally hematogenous in origin, *Staphyloccoccus aureus* is the most common causative pathogen and generally follows skin infection. Age of presentation is commonly 2 to 16 years.

Clinical features vary in infants, children and adults, being related to the structural and vascular differences of bone at these ages. In children older than one year, the epiphyseal plate blocks extension of the infection so the infection spreads laterally into the subperiosteal space or to the joint in which synovial reflections extend beyond the epiphysis to metaphysis, such as the shoulder and hip joints. In infants, small capillaries cross the epiphyseal growth plate, and thus, permit extension of infection to the epiphysis and the joint. In adults, the epiphyseal plate is fused and no longer forms a barrier to the spread of infection from metaphysis to the adjacent joint. Thus acute pyogenic arthritis is a frequent complication of osteomyelitis in infants.

Neonatal osteomyelitis presents with few clinical signs despite multiple sites of involvement, and hence, a complete skeletal survey is warranted in such cases. Premature infants requiring umbilical catheterization are at higher risk for osteomyelitis. Radionuclide bone scintigraphy is advocated in all patients with suspected neonatal osteomyelitis, following initial radiographs.

Plain radiographs are the first imaging study in the work up of osteomyelitis. Soft tissue swelling and small single or multiple osteolytic areas affecting the metaphysis is the earliest change which is seen within 7 to 10 days.

Elevation of the periosteum or periosteal reaction which is lamellar layered new bone formation is seen after 3 to 6 weeks.

Typically, the dead bone (sequestrum) also forms at 3 to 8 weeks. It appears dense. Osteopenia in the surrounding bone due to hyperemia.

Later remodeling reverts the appearance of bone to normal in infants and children but in adults the sclerosis and cortical irregularity persist.

Ultrasonography shows deep soft tissue swelling (earliest sign). Periosteal elevation seen as a hyperechoic line with subperiosteal fluid collection. Cortical breech is seen as focal defect in the cortex. Ultrasonography detects presence of fluid in the joint especially of hip and shoulder joints in an infant.

Radionuclide scintigraphy is the most sensitive investigation for diagnosing acute osteomyelitis 99m Tc labeled methylene diphosphonate (99m Tc-MDP), hydroxymethylene diphosphonate (99m Tc-HMDP) and gallium 67 citrate are the most commonly used radionuclide agents. They show positive findings usually within 3 days and sometimes within 24 hours of onset of infection. Triple phase bone scanning is done, osteomyelitis shows hot areas on all phases.

MRI is an important imaging tool in the evaluation of early osteomyelitis and overlying soft tissue involvement. It is superior to scintigraphy in evaluation of axial skeletal osteomyelitis because of better anatomical delineation. In addition, MRI can distinguish soft tissue infection with periostitis from osteomyelitis.

### Localized Osteomyelitis (Brodie's Abscess)

Localized osteomyelitis or Brodie's abscess is a limited osteomyelitis caused either by organisms of low virulence of high resistance in the host. It occurs most frequently at one end of the bone, but it, may also occur in the diaphysis. It is seen as a well circumscribed osteolytic focus surrounded by a sclerotic margin. Occasionally, a metaphyseal serpiginous channel with sclerotic border marks the tract of infection. This is considered characteristic of nontubercular etiology like *Staphylococcus*, *Streptococcus* or *Hemophilus*. In early stage, when the lesion is small, it is difficult to identify on X-rays and CT or MRI is required.

## CHRONIC OSTEOMYELITIS

Chronic osteomyelitis result from inadequately treated acute osteomyelitis or from infection following compound fracture. Pain, local swelling, discharge from wound, sinus formation, scars and muscle contractures, shortening of bones, deformities and decreased movements and systemic signs and symptoms may be present.

Conventional X-rays show cloacae, involucrum or sequestrum. There are sclerotic and lucent areas admixed with bony thickening and deformities (Fig. 1.14 and Fig. 1.15). In osteomyelitis of the skull, typically no sclerosis is seen.

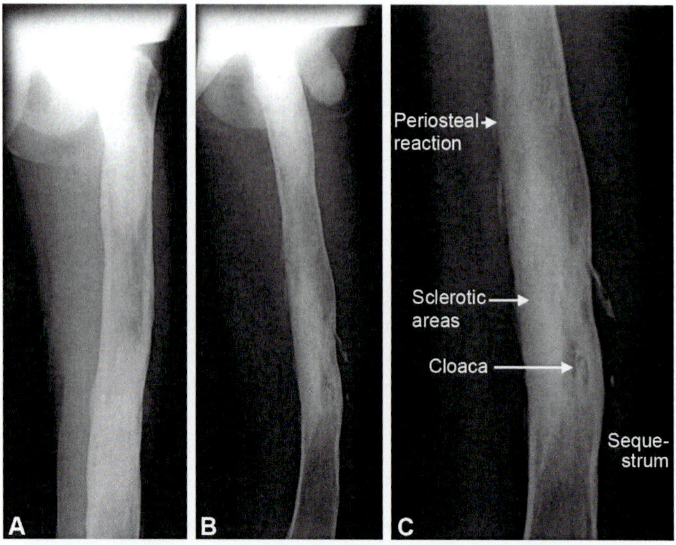


**Figs 1.14A to C:** X-ray thigh shows chronic osteomyelitis. C is magnified view of B

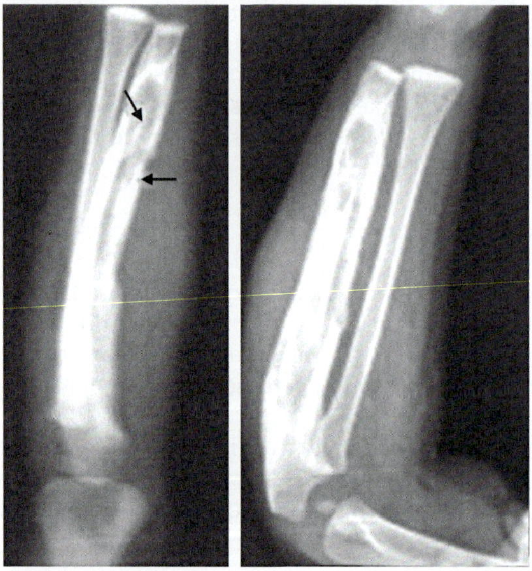

**Fig. 1.15:** X-ray left forearm of a three-year-old male with chronic osteomyelitis, ulna shows cortical thickening, bone destruction and sequestrum formation (arrow)

The sequelae include:

a. Growth plate destruction leading to limb length discrepancy
b. Chronically discharging
c. Extensive bone destruction with modeling deformity
d. Avascular necrosis
e. Pathological fractures
f. Premature osteoarthritis.

Scintigraphy: It is more useful in determining activity. The 67Ga has been recommended as the optimal agent. Following successful treatment 67Ga uptakes should decrease to a normal level.

MRI is used to distinguish regions of active infection from uninvolved marrow or fibrotic regions.

### Sclerosing Osteomyelitis of Garre

A rare type of chronic osteomyelitis occurring in children and young adults, presenting with insidious onset of local pain. There is predilection for involvement of mandible and shafts of long bones.

Radiological appearance is of intense sclerosis resulting in thickened bone. Areas of frank bony destruction are rare. In this, the periosteal reaction and permeative bone destruction are absent.

## SEQUESTRUM

Sequestrum is a piece of dead bone that has become separated during the process of necrosis from normal bone. It is extra dense, more radiopaque and more heavy than surrounding bone. It does not decalcify because of avascularity. Its surface is usually irregular due to erosive process by proteolytic enzymes in granulation tissue.

### Types of Sequestra

1. Tubular or diaphyseal seen in pyogenic osteomyelitis.
2. Trapezoid seen in pyogenic osteomyelitis.
3. Ring seen at end of stumps, around Steinman pin and wires.
4. Flake or feathery seen in tuberculous osteomyelitis in a cavity.
5. Coarse sandy seen in tuberculous osteomyelitis out the cavity.
6. Fine sandy seen in viral osteomyelitis.
7. Black seen in actinomycosis.

## SEPTIC ARTHRITIS

Infectious arthritis affects children and hip joint is a common site to be involved. Spread of infection may be hematogenous, local trauma, neighboring osteomyelitis or adjoining soft tissue infection. Streptococcus Group is frequently implicated. The avascular joint cartilage gets infected through the highly vascular synovial membrane causing edema and effusion, the obliteration of cartilage leads to reduction of joint space and destroys the articular cartilage. Followed by immobilization due to pain leads to osteoporosis and destruction leading to subluxations or dislocations. Other sequelae are fibrous ankylosis and deformity. Initially, radiographs may show joint space widening with soft tissue swelling. Later osteoporosis, loss of joint space, marginal and central erosion of articular cortex is seen (Fig. 1.16).

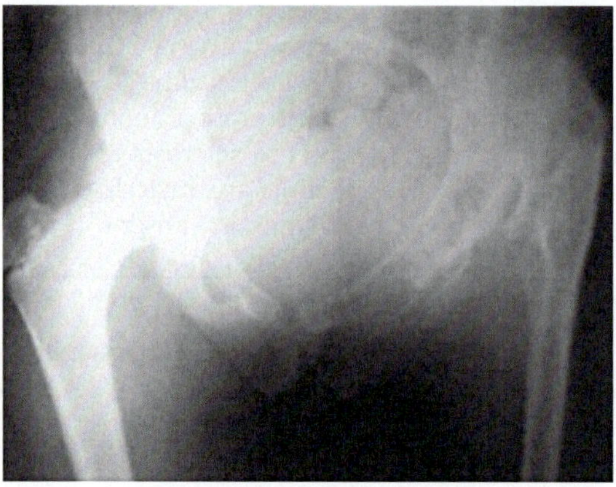

**Fig. 1.16:** Sequelae in septic arthritis left hip in an eight-year-old female in the form of destruction of left femoral head which is displaced superiorly with development of pseudoarthrosis

## PERIOSTEAL REACTION (PERIOSTITIS)

Periosteum is the outer surface of bone which separates bone from surrounding soft tissues. It is firmly adherent to the underlying bone. It is normally not visible on X-rays. An underlying inflammatory or neoplastic process provokes hyperemia that activates fibroblasts to osteoblasts that produce osteoid tissue which gets mineralized and appears as layers of new bone termed as periostitis (Fig 1.17). Presence of periosteal reaction is indicates the biologic underlying process. It takes 10 to 21 days from the initial insult for the periosteal reaction to become visible on X-rays.

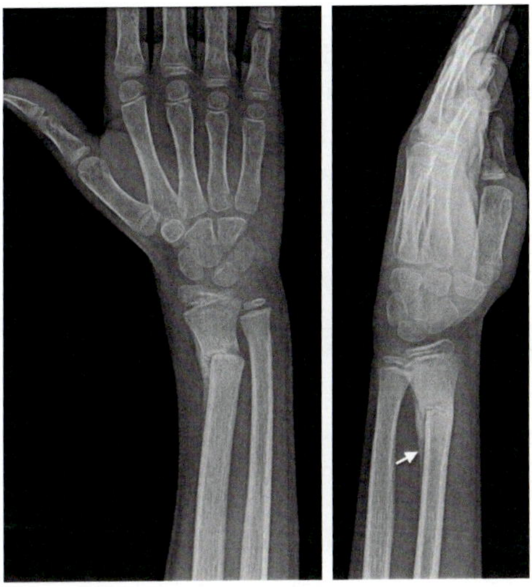

Fig. 1.17: X-ray forearm shows periosteal reaction (arrow) in the process of healing of fracture

## Causes of Periosteal Reaction

i. Trauma
ii. Infection
iii. Inflammatory arthritis
iv. Neoplasm—osteoid osteoma, osteosarcoma, Ewing's sarcoma
v. Congenital—physiological in infants during first 1 to 6 months
vi. Metabolic—hypertrophic pulmonary osteoarthropathy, thyroid acropathy, hypervitaminosis A, fluorosis
vii. Venous insufficiency.

## Types of Periosteal Reaction

a. Continuous—it may be solid, lamellar, multilamellar or parallel spiculated.
   1. Solid—seen as thickening of periosteal surface and indicates benign etiology as in osteoid osteoma, eosinophilic granuloma.
   2. Single lamellar—thin 1 to 2 mm faint radiopaque line from the cortical surface as in histiocytosis, healing fractures.

3. Multilamellar or onion peel—multiple concentric layers of periosteum as in Ewing's sarcoma.
4. Parallel speculated—bony spicules may appear perpendicular to the cortex, i.e. hair on end appearance as seen with thalassemia. Sunburst appearance is due to bony spicules fanning out in focal divergent manner and seen with osteosarcoma.

b. Discontinuous or interrupted mineralization forms an angular configuration with underlying cortex resembling sides of an angle (Codman angles) as in osteogenic sarcoma.
c. Complex reaction includes combination of lamellated, divergent spiculated reaction and Codmans angle.

## TUBERCULOSIS OR CARIES SPINE

Caries spine is the most common form of skeletal tuberculosis constituting 50% of cases. It commonly affects the lower thoracic and lumbar vertebrae mainly due excessive load bearing and mobility of spine in this region and due to presence of large amount of spongy tissue.

Within the vertebra tuberculosis could start in any part and is classified accordingly.

1. Paradiscal/Metaphyseal–most common area involved.
2. Central.
3. Anterior/Periosteal.
4. Appendiceal.
5. Soft tissue extension.

Tuberculosis of spine can occur at any age but most patients are under thirty years of age. Some patients may be asymptomatic, afebrile, others present with constitutional symptoms. Usual presentation is persistent back pain, local tenderness and limitation of spinal mobility. Paraparesis may be early onset in about 20%, which develops during the active phase usually due to cord compression by epidural abscess, pathological subluxation. Late onset paraplegia can occur due to dural fibrosis, severe kyphoscoliotic deformity, spinal canal stenosis, gliosis of cord and cord infarction due to endarteritis.

### Diagnosis

Laboratory investigation show anemia, lymphocytosis, hypoproteinemia and raised ESR.

### *X-ray Spine*

i. Early stage shows disk space narrowing to loss of disk space and reduced bone density
ii. Late stage shows anterior wedging (compression) of vertebral body in case of anterior vertebral type.

Central vertebral body collapse/concertina collapse (central type). Destruction of posterior elements (appendiceal type).

Soft tissue swelling and its calcification are highly suggestive of tuberculosis. vertebral body and posterior elements appear more dense due to sclerosis.

Paravertebral shadow on X-ray indicates cold abscess.

CT identifies paravertebral soft tissue swelling more readily than X-rays. It helps to assess the degree of neural compromise.

MRI—it helps in further delineation of the disease (Figs 1.18A to D) and help to detect cord compromise.

CT and MRI—detect involvement of posterior spinal elements, craniovertebral and craniodorsal region, sacrum and sacroiliac region.

Gallium scanning—it is useful in disseminated TB.

USG is useful to detect size of cold abscess in lumbar vertebral disease.

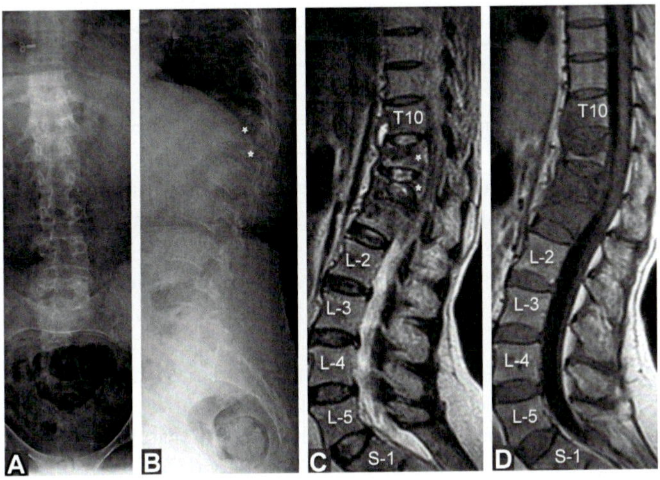


**Figs 1.18A to D:** (A and B) X-ray AP and lateral view dorsolumbar spine shows anterior wedging of D11 vertebral body (inferior asterisk) with partial destruction of D11 and the disks D11-D12 and D12-L1; (C and D) MRI confirms the X-ray findings, shows vertebral destruction of D11 to L1 involving the intervening disks. There is a small anterior paraspinal abscess

## BENIGN AND MALIGNANT BONE TUMOR

Bone tumors present radiological image which may be simple to diagnose like bone cyst, fibrous dysplasia or osteogenic sarcoma or may be very difficult to diagnose. Primary malignant tumors of bone are responsible for only one percent of all deaths from neoplasia. More common for malignancy in bones is metastatic rather than primary. Radiology serves not only to provide a diagnosis but also to delineate soft tissue and extend of bony involvement (Table 1.2).

**Table 1.2** Differentiation between benign and malignant bone tumor

| Benign Tumors | Malignant Tumors |
|---|---|
| Slow growing | Rapid growth |
| Asymptomatic, few symptoms | Pain, swelling, joint movement limitation |
| Well circumscribed margins, narrow transition zone | Ill defined margins, zone of transition is wide |
| Noninvading | Invasion is seen into soft tissues |
| No metastasis | Metastasizes |
| X-ray shows a lytic or sclerotic lesion with corticated margins, no soft tissue extension is seen | X-ray shows aggressive lytic or mixed density lesion with cortical break, soft tissue extension is present |

## UNICAMERAL OR SIMPLE BONE CYST

Unicameral bone cyst or simple bone cyst is an seen in the first two decades of life with M:F ratio of 2:1. It is situated in the metaphysis of the long bones commonly upper end of humerus or upper end of femur.

There are two types of cyst (1) Active cyst is situated close to the epiphyseal plate (2) Inactive or latent cyst when the cyst has moved away from the growth plate.

The bone cyst is generally asymptomatic. Pain may occur if a pathological fracture takes place. Joint deformities like shortening, lengthening, coxa vara, coxa valga may occur due to proximity of cyst to the growth plate.

On plain X-ray, it appears as a well defined lytic lesion with sclerotic borders located at the metaphysis which moves to the diaphysis as age advances. Overlying cortex is thinned out with or without cortical breach. Fallen fragment sign is due to fractured cyst when a piece of the bone migrates into the cavity and settles at the base. CT and MRI depict this signs better but patient should be subjective to CT and MRI only in equivocal cases.

Surgical excision is the treatment of choice. However curettage and bone grafting, subtotal resection and bone grafting and total resection and bone grafting is also carried out.

## OSTEOID OSTEOMA

Osteoid osteoma is a benign lesion frequently found in the appendicular skeleton. The tumors produce excess bone and secrete pain-causing prostaglandins, resulting in intense pain especially at night. A 17-year-old male presented with pain and tenderness in left thigh region since 4 months. Radiograph shows sclerosis and cortical thickening due to subperiosteal bone formation. The radiolucent nidus is questionably visualized. The location of the nidus, intranidal calcification, sclerosis, mature periosteal bone formation and location of original cortex is precisely demonstrated by CT. MRI also clearly showed the partially calcified nidus and associated cortical thickening. In addition, MR images revealed mild marrow and soft tissue edema in the vicinity of the nidus, which is not demonstrated by CT (Figs 1.19A to E).

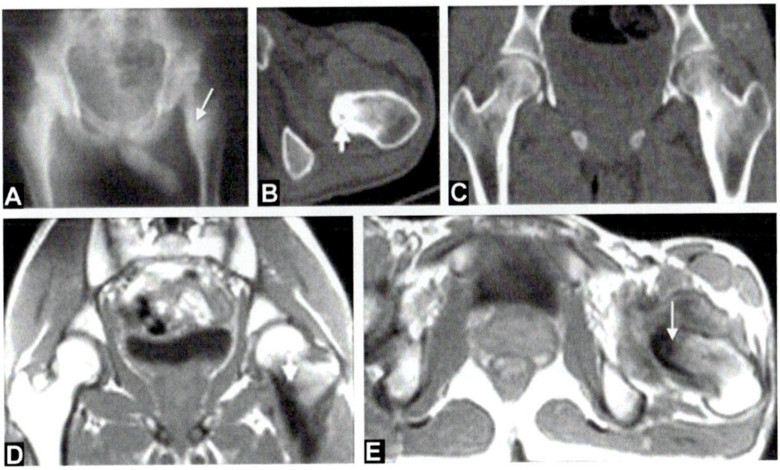


**Figs 1.19A to E:** Plain radiograph of 17-year-old male shows (A) an ill-defined region of increased cortical thickness (arrow) and CT axial (B) and coronal reformatted (C) reveals the presence of small well defined calcified nidus and dense cortical thickening near lesser trochanter. MRI coronal (D) and axial (E) reveals hypointense cortical thickening along lesser trochanter with well defined small hypointense lesion adjacent to it (arrow)

## OSTEOCHONDROMA

Osteochondroma is also known as *exostosis*. It is the most common benign bone tumor seen in children and young adults. It has its origin from metaphysis with cartilage cap covering and bony attachment to underlying host bone. It is located at the sites of tendinous attachment around the metaphysis of long bones in the region of knee, ankle, hip, shoulder and elbow.

Patient is usually asymptomatic but may complain of pain, swelling, pathological fracture commonly secondary to complications. Clinical examination reveals a firm nontender swelling fixed to the bone around joints and decreased joint movements. Multiple osteochondromas occur as a manifestation of diaphyseal aclasia.

X-ray shows a sessile or pedunculated outgrowth of bone at the metaphysis, cortical and medullary portions of which are continuous with the parent bone. It usually points away from the joint (Fig. 1.20). CT and MRI can clearly depict the continuity of the marrow and cortex of host bone into osteochondroma. Malignant transformation into low grade chondrosarcoma occurs in 1% cases.

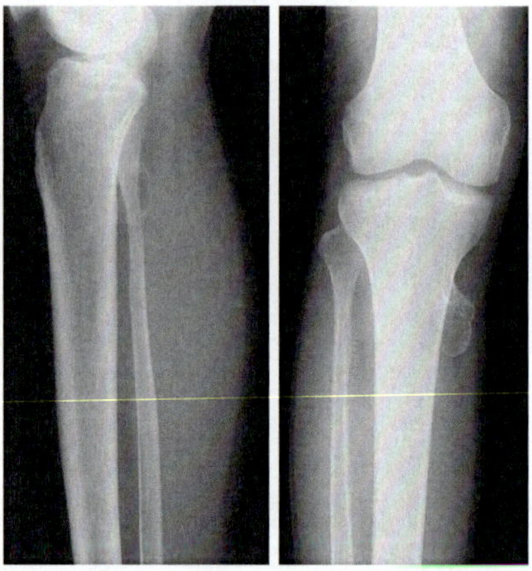

**Fig. 1.20:** X-ray leg shows pedunculated (arrow) osteochondroma seen arising from medial surface of proximal tibia

Indication for surgical excision is pathological fracture, limitation of joint movements and malignant transformation.

## OSTEOCHONDROMA RIB

It has been estimated that rib osteochondromas arise in almost 50% of patients with multiple hereditary exostoses. The rib exostoses that project externally are palpable on the chest wall. Osteochondromas can mimic pulmonary nodules. CT is most helpful in determining the nature of these bone growths (Fig. 1.21).

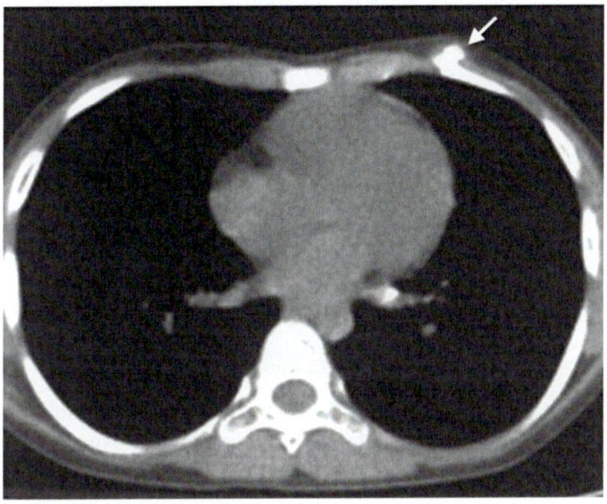

Fig. 1.21: Osteochondroma (arrow) in a 10-year-old female child arising from the anterior end of left rib

## ADAMANTINOMA

Adamantinoma is a rare tumor typically involving the midshaft of tibia. Its pathogenesis is unknown but is histologically similar to ameloblastoma of the jaw. Most cases occur between 10 and 50 yrs of age. Male to female ratio is 5:4. Local pain and tenderness of several months to years is the most common presenting complaint. More than 90% occur in the tibia mostly in the midshaft. Other bones involved are fibula, ulna and femur.

Plain radiograph shows central or eccentric osteolytic lesion in the shaft of the bone with well defined margin, causing mild expansion of the bone (Fig. 1.22). Multiloculated appearance and satellite lesion are useful diagnostic features. Periosteal reaction is uncommon. It grows at slow rate but is characterized by local recurrences and metastasis to lungs. Extensive local resection is the usual form of treatment.

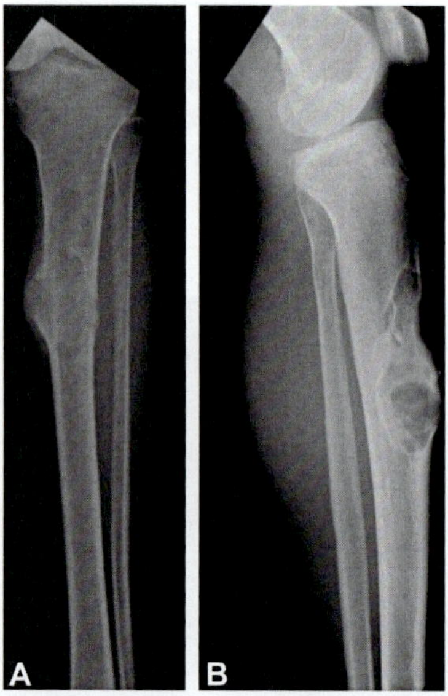

**Figs 1.22A and B:** AP and lateral X-rays of left leg show eccentric multiloculated osteolytic lesion in the tibial shaft with well defined margin causing expansion of the bone

### Ameloblastoma

Ameloblastoma is benign locally aggressive epithelial neoplasm also known as adamantinoma of jaw. It originates from enamel type epithelial tissue element around tooth. It occurs in 3rd to 5th decade of life. It is located in the ramus and posterior body of mandible in the region of angle of mandible.

On imaging, it manifest as a well defined, well corticated, unilocular or multilocular lytic expansile lesion giving soap bubble or honeycomb appearance. It shows tendency of local recurrence after resection.

## GIANT CELL TUMOR

Giant cell tumor (GCT) is usually a benign typically found in the metaepiphysis of long bones. It is locally aggressive tumor originates from undifferentiated cells of supporting tissues of bone marrow and is commonly occurs in young adults at 20 to 30 years of age. Tumor arises eccentrically in the metaphysis with tendency to approach subarticular cortex as they enlarge. Seventy to eighty percent occurs in the lower end of femur, upper end of tibia, fibula and distal end of radius.

Clinically presents as swelling near the joint on one side. Tenderness is moderate or absent. Egg shell crackling sensation may be present. There may be pathological fracture and limitation of joint movements in late stage.

Types are:

a. Benign GCT (more common)
b. Malignant GCT

X-ray (Fig. 1.23) shows well defined multiloculated osteolytic lesion which expands the overlying cortex (soap bubble appearance) with no surrounding sclerosis (85% cases). It may be associated with soft tissue component. Periosteal reaction is uncommon. MRI is best modality to diagnose recurrence following treatment. Pathological fracture may be present.

### Treatment

1. On surgery en block excision is the procedure of choice.
2. Curettage and bone grafting, curettage and acrylic cementation or cryosurgery. Excision and reconstruction.
3. Radiotherapy for surgically inaccessible or inoperable tumor.
4. Amputation is done for widespread aggressive lesion.

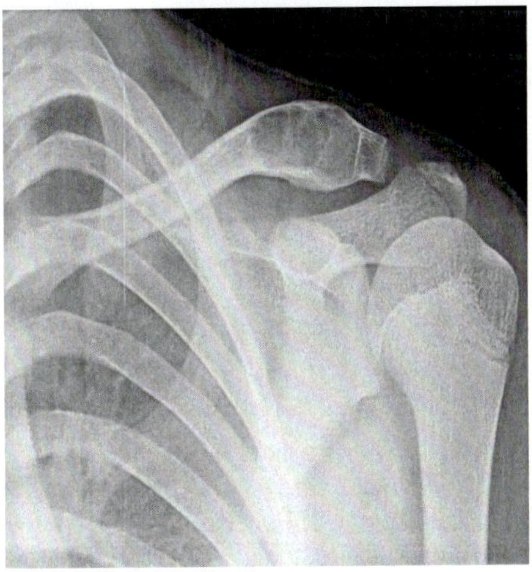

**Fig. 1.23:** X-ray shoulder PA view shows well defined expansile lytic lesion involving lateral third of the clavicle suggestive of GCT, other differential is aneurysmal bone cyst

## SKELETAL METASTASIS

Primary tumors which originate in other organs and involve the skeletal structures of the body either by hematogenous, lymphatic route or by direct invasion are called metastasis. Metastasis are generally multiple commonly found in the axial skeleton and sites of residual red marrow. It is the most common tumor of the bone. The common sites are vertebrae, pelvic bones, proximal femora and humerii, skull and ribs (Figs 1.24A to C). It is unusual for metastasis to involve bones distal to the elbows or knees.

The common primary neoplasm which spread to bones is carcinoma of breast, lungs, prostate, kidney and thyroid.

Occult primary is a primary malignancy in which there are no localizing signs suggestive of the site of primary tumor and has not been detected by any of the available investigative protocols. However, the metastatic lesions have been detected on clinical, radiological and biomedical parameters. Histopathology may suggest the likely site of primary.

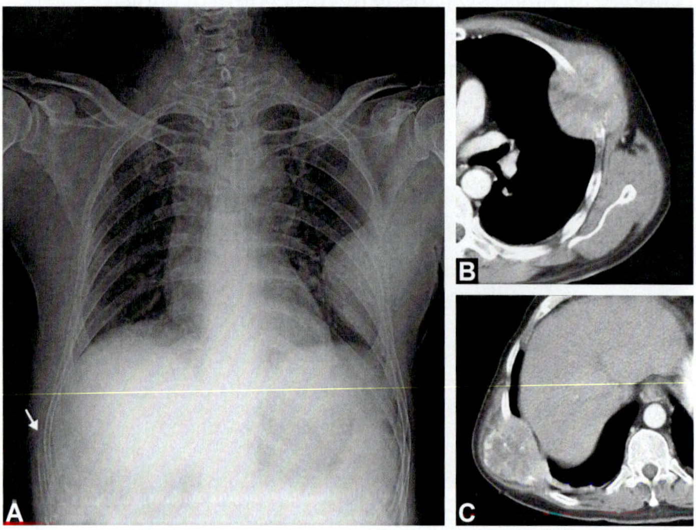


**Figs 1.24A to C:** X-ray chest (A) shows a large (8 × 6 cm) well defined mass lesion abutting the left lower chest wall with broad base towards the chest wall with partial destruction lateral aspect 4th rib on the left. Contrast CT chest shows moderately enhancing metastatic bone lesion which is rounded well defined having a large soft tissue component from the left 4th rib (B) and right 10th rib (C) laterally, the ribs are partially destroyed, few small scattered calcific densities are seen in the lesions

## DIAPHYSEAL ACLASIS

X-ray chest shows a large bony outgrowth-exostosis arising from superior medial aspect of right scapula; it is not possible to say if this large exostosis is pedunculated or sessile. Another exostosis is seen to arise from medial margin of upper shaft of left humerus and another small bony outgrowth from the lateral margin of upper 3rd shaft of right humerus (Fig. 1.25). On CT chest, the origin of lesion can be best evaluated (Fig. 1.26).

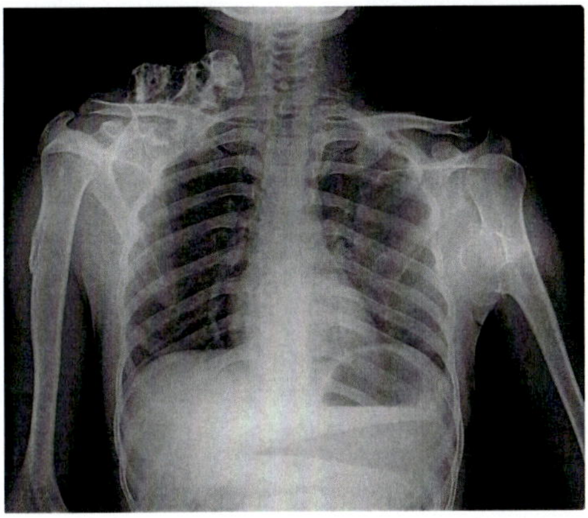

Fig. 1.25: Diaphyseal aclasis

On CT chest coronal reconstruction, a large exostosis is seen to arise from the anterosuperior margin of right scapula (Fig. 1.26). The exostosis has a pedicle which was not appreciated on PA chest, is clearly seen on CT.

Diaphyseal aclasis is also known as external chondromatosis syndrome, multiple exostoses, or multiple osteochondromatosis. Usually presents during the first decade of life. It is characterized by multiple exostosis or bony protrusions and is inherited autosomal dominant disorder. Long bones are usually affected more severely and more frequently than the short bones but they also often involve the medial borders of the scapulae, ribs and iliac crests. The malignant change is more frequent compared to the solitary exostosis. Most of the osteochondromas are painless and the main concern is often cosmetic.

Plain X-ray may be the only imaging study required. CT scan is useful in the assessment of osteochondromas in the pelvis, shoulder or spine. MRI scan is useful in the assessment of malignant transformation and for evaluating compression of the spinal cord, nerve roots and peripheral nerves.

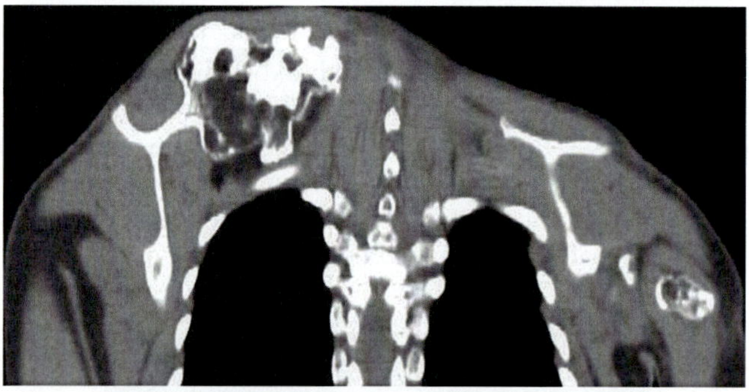

**Fig. 1.26:** CT chest shows diaphyseal aclasis

## PREAXIAL AND POSTAXIAL POLYDACTYLY

Polydactyly may be preaxial (radial) or postaxial (ulnar). It may range from an ossicle to complete duplication of fingers or toes. On occasion the hand may be duplicated. When present, should search for an associated syndrome. Syndactyly may be associated with polydactyly. Postaxial polydactyly is more frequent and often seen as fifth digit duplications in hands or feet (Figs 1.27A to D).

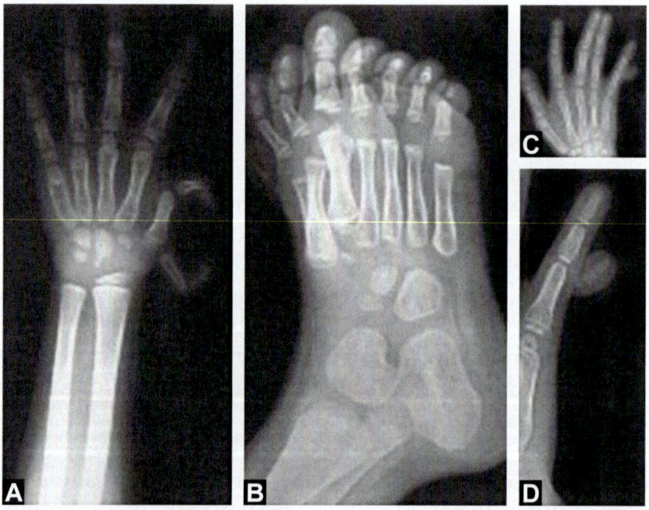


**Figs 1.27A to D:** (A) AP radiograph of hand shows pre-axial (radial) polydactyly in a six-year-old female; (B) Oblique radiograph of foot shows pre-axial polydactyly in 14-year-old male; (C) Shows post-axial (ulnar) polydactyly; (D) It is magnified view of C

## ECTRODACTYLY ECTODERMAL DYSPLASIA CLEFT LIP (EEC) SYNDROME

Ectrodactyly ectodermal dysplasia cleft lip (EEC) syndrome is a uncommon condition with multiple congenital anomalies with normal intelligence characterized by ectodermal dysplasia, clefting of hands, feet, lip and palate. It is an autosomal dominant syndrome. Management of the cases requires a multidisciplinary approach. Early diagnosis allows precise counseling of parents with reassurance of normal intelligence.

Examination of the baby revealed ectrodactyly (splitting of hands and feet), ectodermal dysplasia, cleft lip and palate, sparse scalp hairs and eyebrows and absence of eye lashes.

These abnormalities constitute the EEC syndrome (Figs 1.28A to E).

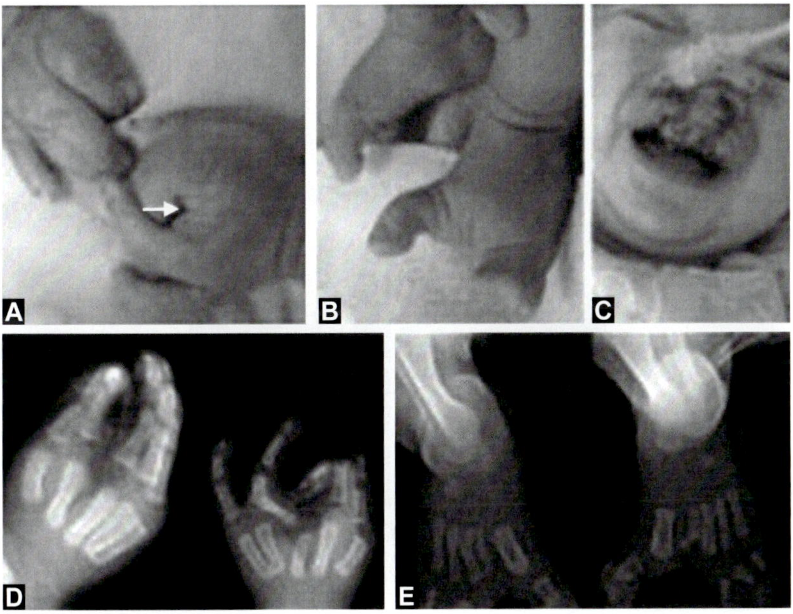


**Figs 1.28A to E:** Both hands have claw like appearance due to cone shaped defect (arrow). Soft tissue fusion of the middle and ring finger of the right hand and index and middle finger of the left hand is seen (A) Both feet show claw like appearance due to soft tissue fusion of the 3rd, 4th and 5th toes; (B) Surgery has been performed for cleft lip; (C) X-ray hands; (D) show a cone-shaped defect. There is absence of middle and distal phalanges of middle finger on the left side; (E) X-ray feet show cone shaped defect due to absence of 2nd toe on either side. Syndactyly of the metatarsals of the left foot is seen. There is absence of middle and distal phalanges of 3rd, 4th and 5th toes on either side

## MADELUNG'S DEFORMITY

Madelung's deformity is common in girls and is generally bilateral and presents during adolescence. The defective development of the inner third of the epiphysis of the lower end of the radius results in bowing of radial shaft thus increasing the interosseous space. The lower end of ulna is subluxed backward. The hand projects forward at the wrist joint to produce a bayonet-like appearance in a lateral projection (Fig. 1.29).

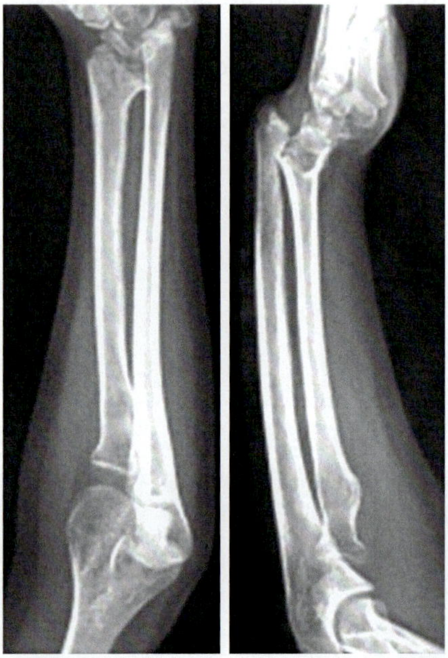

**Fig. 1.29:** Madelung's deformity of right wrist in a 13-year-old female

## CONGENITAL HIP DISLOCATION

Congenital hip dislocation is a very important condition as treatment depends upon early recognition. Females are more commonly affected (F>M, 5:1). Dislocation is usually unilateral (L>R, 11:1), both hips may be involved. Ultrasound is now the accepted method of primary investigation of suspected developmental dysplasia of the hip (Fig. 1.30).

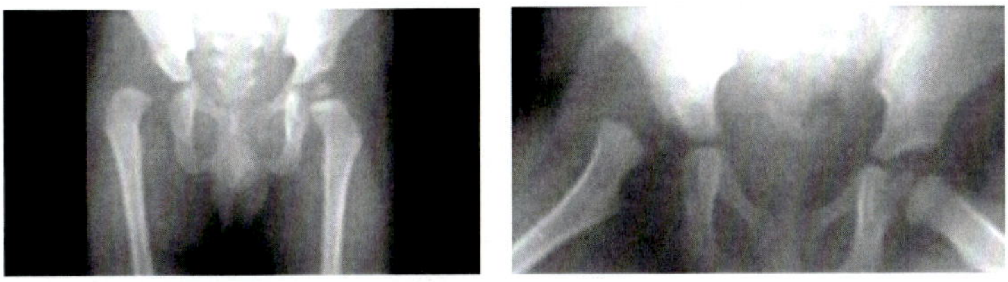

Fig. 1.30: AP and frog pelvis radiographs shows congenital hip dislocation in a 3-year-old male

## MULTIPLE EPIPHYSEAL DYSPLASIA

It is characterized by an abnormality of mucopolysaccharoid and glycoprotein metabolism and develops in early childhood. Radiographs show delayed ossification and delayed mineralization of the epiphysis of long bones which are fragmented small and flattened, loose bodies may also occur in joints (Fig. 1.31). Metaphyseal irregularity is seen in tubular bones, when spine is involved there is irregularity of vertebral endplates.

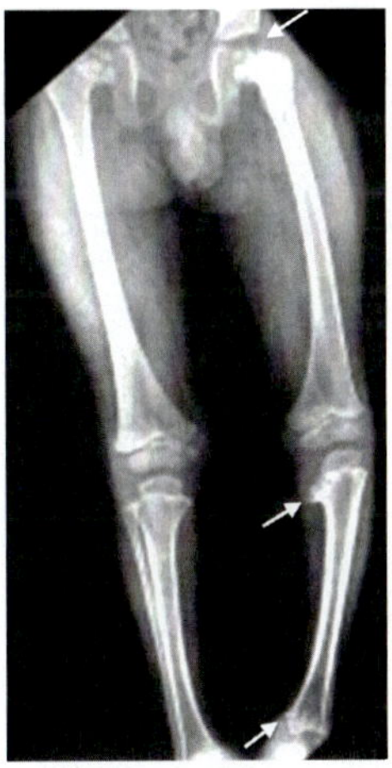

Fig. 1.31 A 5-year-old male with multiple epiphyseal dysplasia shows bilateral involvement of long bones of lower limbs

## MACRODYSTROPHIA LIPOMATOSA

Macrodystrophia lipomatosa is a congenital local gigantism of the hand and foot, characterized by proliferation of all mesenchymal components, particularly fibroadipose tissue (Figs 1.32A to C and 1.33A and B). Macrodystrophia lipomatosa comes to clinical attention because of cosmetic reasons, mechanical problems secondary to degenerative joint disease or development of neurovascular compression.

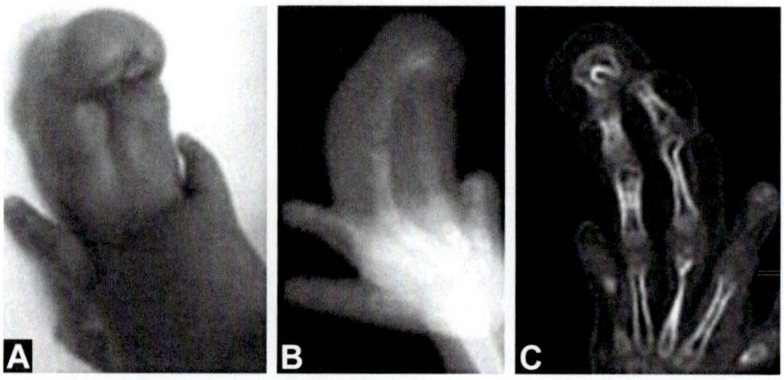

**Figs 1.32A to C** (A) Clinical photograph of right hand shows enlarged, fused ring and middle finger; (B) Plain radiograph; (C) coronal reformatted CT shows soft tissue swelling and proliferation of fat on palmar aspect of the ring and middle fingers, along with dorsal angulation and syndactyly

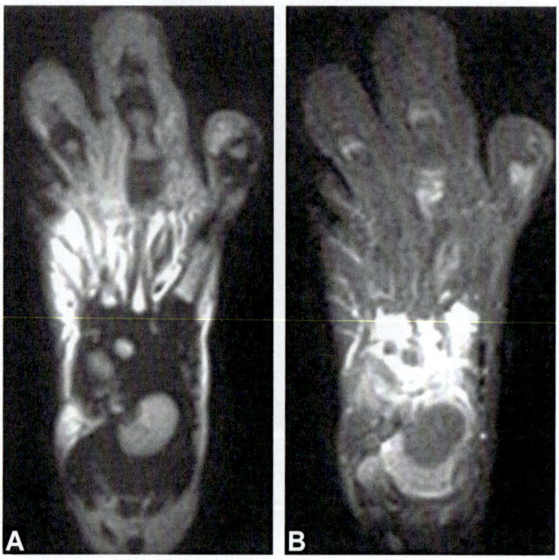

**Figs 1.33A and B:** T1 coronal MRI (A) reveals proliferation of fatty tissue on plantar aspect of the second and third toes of right foot with signal intensity similar to that of subcutaneous fat as seen by fat suppressed STIR coronal image (B)

## HOLT-ORAM SYNDROME

Holt-Oram syndrome is an inherited disorder that causes abnormalities of the hands, arms, spine and heart. Occurs approximately in one in every 100,000 and affects both sexes equally.

It falls into two groups: (1) Defects in arm and hand bones involving one or both sides of the body. Most commonly the defects are in the carpal bones and thumb. The thumb may be malformed or missing. In severe cases, the arms may be very short such that the hands are attached close to the body (phocomelia). (2) Heart abnormalities. Three-fourth of cases with Holt-Oram syndrome have heart abnormality. It may be abnormal rhythms, atrial or ventricular septal defect (Figs 1.34A to D).

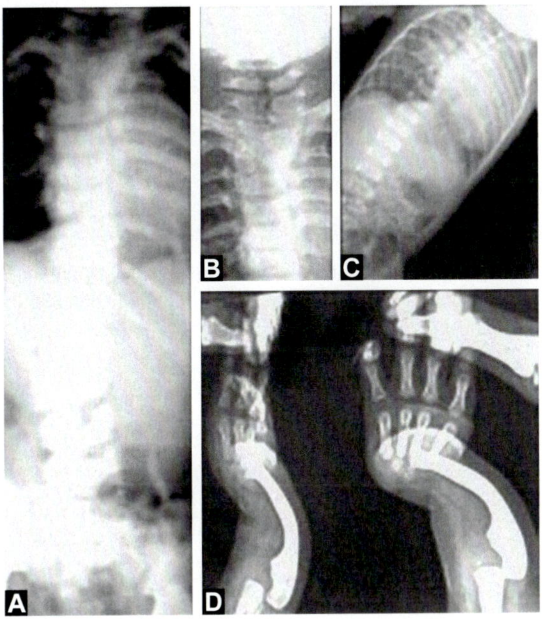

**Figs 1.34A to D:** (A and B) X-rays of spine show multiple spinal anomalies; (C) shows congenital heart disease; (D) shows absence of radius. All these are features of Holt-Oram syndrome

## OSTEONECROSIS OF HIP (LEGG-CALVE-PERTHES DISEASE)

Perthes is a self-limiting disease seen between 3 to 12 years of age, more common in boys. Patient presents with a limp. The underlying pathology is vascular occlusive episodes of femoral head; the ossific nucleus of the epiphysis suffers necrosis causing growth arrest. Cartilage overlying the femoral head thickens followed by remodeling. Plain radiographs show growth retardation with reduced size of capital femoral epiphysis, subchondral fissuring and fractures and increased density of ossific nucleus. The amount of subchondral fissuring of the femoral head during the initial stages is thought to have prognostic predictive value, the prognosis is poor when associated with more than 50% subchondral fissuring (Figs 1.35A and B).

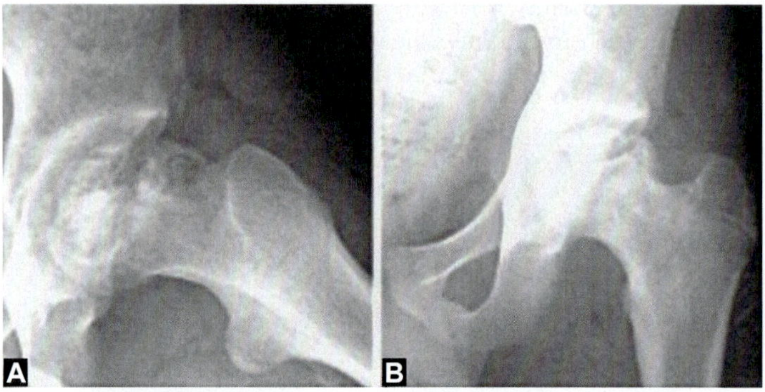


**Figs 1.35A and B:** (A) X-ray left hip shows reduced size and subchondral fissuring of capital femoral epiphysis; (B) shows reduced size, fissuring, fragmentation and increased density of capital femoral epiphysis

# 2 CHAPTER

# Chest

**Chapter Outline**

- Anatomy of Chest and Mediastinum
- Consolidation
- Pleural Effusion
- Pulmonary Tuberculosis
- Miliary Tuberculosis
- Pneumoconiosis
- Pneumothorax
- Aspergilloma/Fungal Ball
- Hydatid Cyst
- Flail Chest
- Kartagener's Syndrome
- Tumors of the Lung
- Pancoast Tumor
- Solitary Pulmonary Nodule or Coin Lesion
- Hamartoma
- Multiple Pulmonary Nodules

## ANATOMY OF CHEST AND MEDIASTINUM

Application of chest CT has greatly increased over the years, however chest radiography remains the most frequently requisitioned and performed imaging examination. A good understanding of normal anatomy and variations is essential for the interpretation of chest radiographs.

On postero-anterior (PA) view (Fig. 2.1), the X-ray beam first enters the patient from the back and then passes through the patient to the film that is placed anterior to the patient's chest. It uses 80-120 kVp and focus film distance of 6 feet. On a PA film, lung is divided radiologically into three zones (Fig. 2.2):

1. Upper zone extends from apices to lower border of 2nd rib anteriorly.
2. Middle zone extends from the lower border of 2nd rib anteriorly to lower border of 4th rib anteriorly.

3. Lower zone extends from the lower border of 4th rib anteriorly to lung bases.

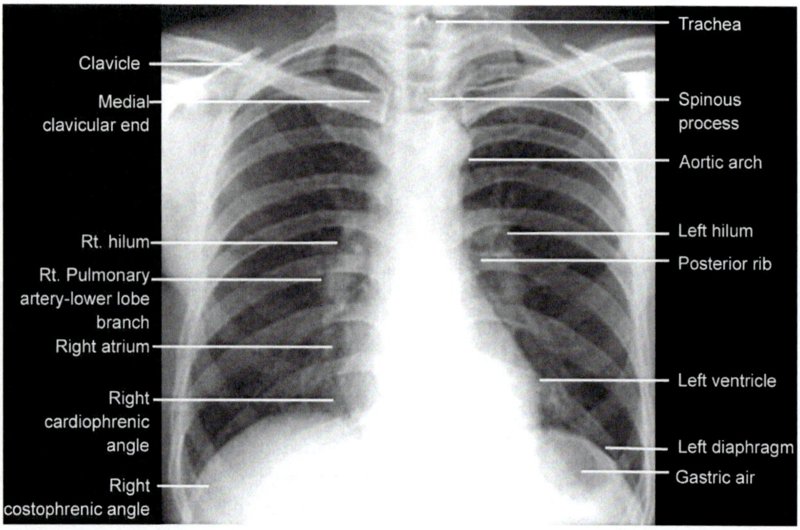


**Fig. 2.1:** Chest X-ray PA view

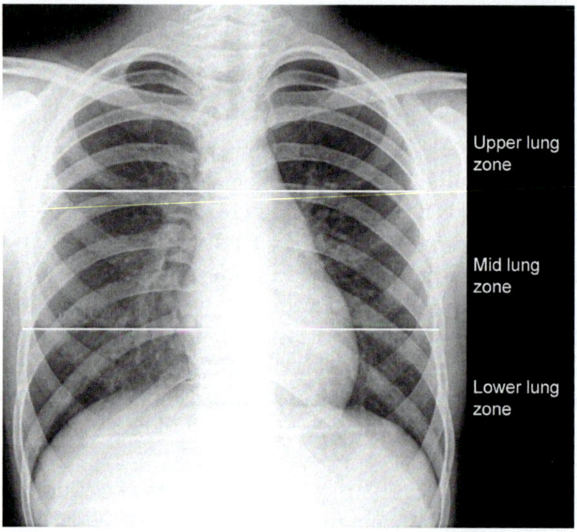


**Fig. 2.2:** Chest X-ray PA view shows lung zones

Radiological division does not depict anatomical lobes of the lung.

In a well centered chest X-ray, medial ends of clavicles are equidistant from vertebral spinous process. Lung fields are of equal density.

Horizontal fissure might be seen on the right side as a thin white line that runs from right hilum to sixth rib laterally. For a fissure to be seen on a radiograph, the X-ray beam has to be tangential to it.

The most frequently observed accessory fissure is the azygos lobe fissure which is seen in 1% of people. It is a normal variant found in the right lung; separated from the upper lobe by a deep pleural furrow housing the azygos vein. It is a small lobe of no clinical significance and hence requires no treatment.

It forms when the azygos vein fails to migrate to the apex of the lung but courses through the lung during fetal life, drawing with it the parietal and visceral pleura. These four layers of pleura form the azygos fissure, and the lung tissue separated from the rest of the lung is called the azygos lobe. As a result, the azygos vein comes to lie at the bottom of a deep fissure in the upper lobe of the right lung. Chest X-ray (Fig. 2.3) shows upside down comma shaped azygos vein lying at the lower medial end of the azygos fissure.

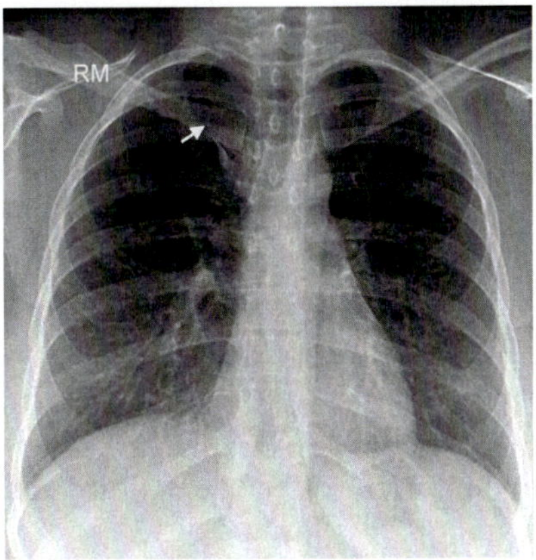


**Fig. 2.3:** Azygos lobe and fissure (arrow)

Both hila are concave outwards. The pulmonary arteries, upper lobe veins and bronchi contribute to the making of hilar shadows. The left hilum is slightly higher than right hilum.

The normal length of trachea is 10 cm, it is central in position and bifurcates at T4-T5 vertebral level. Left atrial enlargement increases the tracheal bifurcation angle (normal is 60°). An inhaled foreign body is likely to lodge in the right lung due to the fact that the right main bronchus is shorter, straighter and wider than left.

Normal heart shadow is uniformly white with maximum transverse diameter less than half of the maximum transthoracic diameter. Cardiothoracic ratio is estimated from the PA view of chest (Fig. 2.5). It is the ratio between the maximum transverse diameter of the heart and the maximum width of thorax above the costophrenic angles: a = right heart border to midline, b = left heart border to midline, c = maximum thoracic diameter above costophrenic angles from inner borders of ribs. Cardiothoracic ratio = a + b: c. Normal cardiothoracic ratio is less than 1:2.

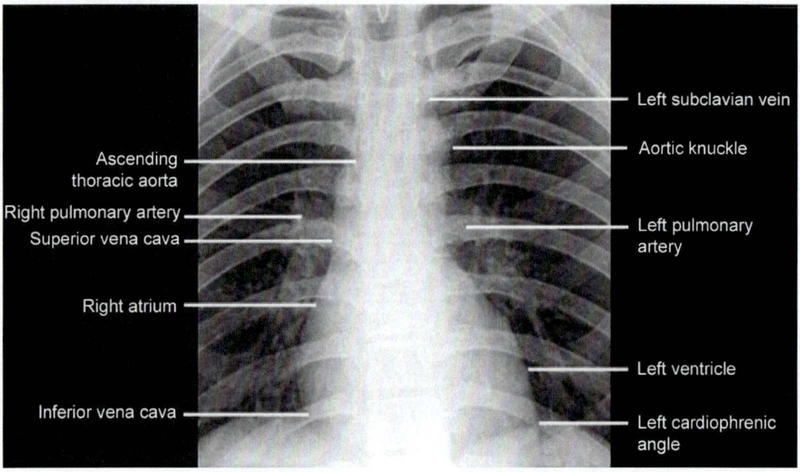


**Fig. 2.4:** Mediastinal border on X-ray chest PA view

Borders of the mediastinum are sharp and distinct (Fig. 2.4). The right heart border is formed by superior vena cava superiorly and right atrium inferiorly, the left heart border is formed by the aortic knuckle superiorly, left atrial appendage and left ventricle inferiorly.

Right hemidiaphragm is higher than left. Costophrenic angles are acute angles.

To detect any pulmonary pathology it is important to remember the normal thoracic architecture, both lungs are compared for areas of abnormal opacities, translucency or uneven bronchovascular distribution in the lungs.

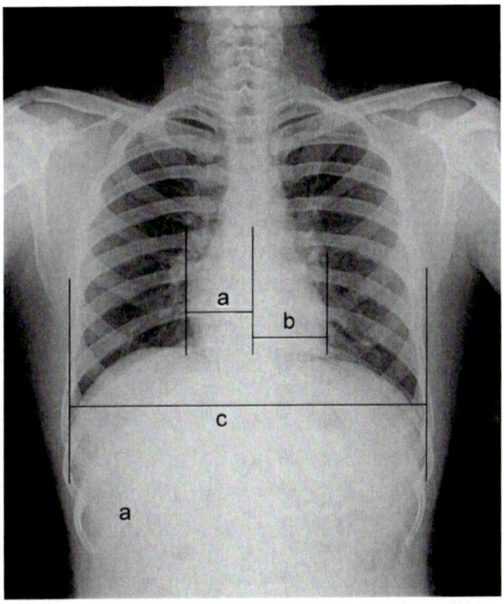


Fig. 2.5: X-ray chest PA view shows cardiothoracic ratio

An abnormal opacity should be closely studied to ensure that it is not amalgamated opacity formed by superimposed normal structures such as bones, costal cartilages, vessels, muscles or nipple. Any opacity is evaluated by its extent, margins and location with presence or absence of calcification or cavitations. A general assessment survey is made to look for any other lesion or displacement of adjacent structures.

## CONSOLIDATION

Acinus is the smallest functional unit of the lung comprising of respiratory bronchioles, alveolar ducts, alveolar sacs and alveoli. When air in acini is replaced by fluid, it is termed as consolidation. This fluid may spread between adjacent acini due to communication between terminal airways producing larger confluent areas of radiopacity which can be appreciated on chest X-ray as a white shadow.

But few airways which still have some air appear black. Hence, in a focus of consolidation, air (black) is seen amidst the fluid/cells in alveolar space (white) giving rise to air-bronchogram. Air Bronchogram sign (by Fleischner) is seen in consolidation, pulmonary edema, hyaline membrane disease, lymphoma and sarcoidosis.

Consolidation may be due to:

a. Infections-bacterial *Staphylococcus aureus, Streptococcus pneumoniae, Klebsiella, Mycobacterial tuberculosis, Mycoplasma pneumoniae* or *Pneumocystis carinii*
b. Neoplasms-bronchogenic carcinoma, lymphoma
c. Acute respiratory distress syndrome
d. Traumatic contusion.

On imaging it appears as a homogeneously increased opacity in the segmental or lobar distribution with or without air bronchogram within it. It may be limited by fissures. There is no loss of lung volume in contrast to atelectasis where increased opacity is associated with loss of lung volume. With treatment density reduces as air returns.

Radiological consolidation may lag behind clinical pneumonia in early phase. Radiological resolution of consolidation lags behind the clinical signs. Hence, X-ray should be repeated at least 2 weeks of proper treatment. Non-resolution of the consolidation for 3 weeks even after appropriate medical therapy should raise possibility of malignant etiology as the underlying cause.

Complication of pneumonia can be:

a. Pleural effusion and empyema
b. Hydropneumothorax
c. Abscess formation
d. Bronchiectasis.

When a part of lung that is adjacent to heart, e.g. the right middle lobe or lingula (Fig. 2.6) is consolidated then its density becomes same as that

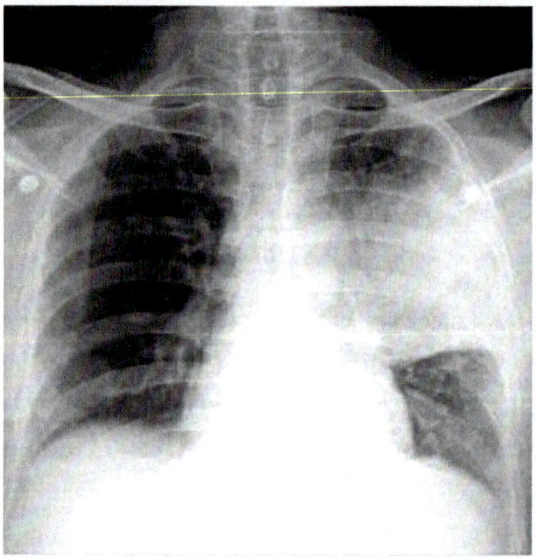

**Fig. 2.6:** Consolidation lingular segment left upper lobe

of heart and merges with it so that it cannot be seen separately from heart and this is called-the Silhouette sign (by Felson). Right middle lobe and lingular pathology obliterates the adjacent heart border.

## PLEURAL EFFUSION

Pleural effusion is the accumulation of fluid in the pleural space, i.e. between the visceral and parietal layers of pleura. The fluid may be transude, exudate (Table 2.1), blood, chyle or rarely bile.

Imaging modalities used are X-ray, USG and CT scan. On chest X-ray pleural effusion is seen as a homogenous opacification with concave upper margin (*meniscus sign*) on erect film (Fig. 2.7) in the lower zone with blunting of costophrenic angle and diaphragm (Fig. 2.7). A massive effusion leads to complete opacification of the hemithorax with contralateral mediastinal shift. Pleural fluid may loculate due to adhesions (Fig. 2.8A). Loculation within the fissure gives appearance of a pseudotumor (Fig. 2.8B). Lateral decubitus view is the most sensitive to detect small pleural effusion (as small as 10 to 50 ml).

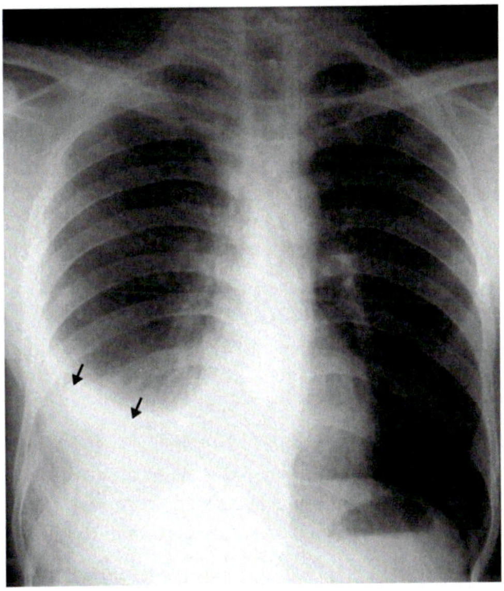

Fig. 2.7: Chest X-ray shows pleural effusion on right side (arrows)

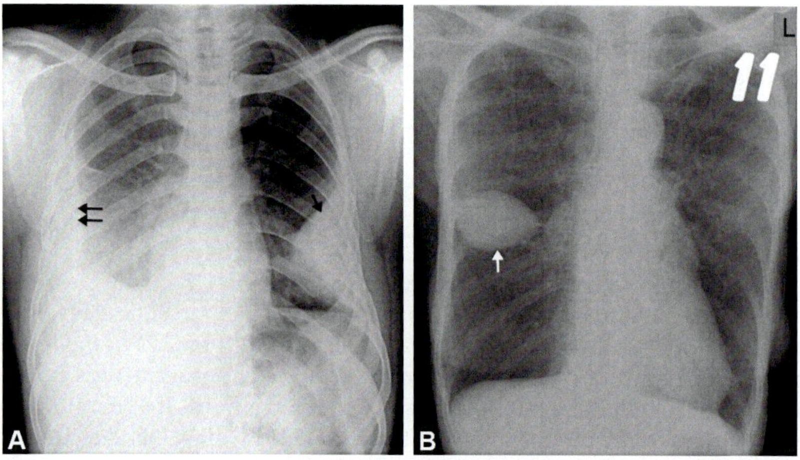


**Figs 2.8A and B:** (A) Chest X-ray shows encysted effusion (arrow) along left lateral chest wall, on right there is free pleural effusion (twin arrow); (B) Loculation of fluid within the lesser fissure (white arrow) on right side gives appearance of a pseudotumor

USG chest confirms the presence or absence of the pleural fluid; it also shows the septations within the pleural fluid with or without solid component within the lesion. USG helps in guiding aspiration of pleural fluid.

CT scan is the most sensitive modality for detection of presence of minimal fluid. It allows distinction between free and loculated fluid showing it's extend and localization.

**Table 2.1:** Distinction between transudate and exudate

| Transudate | Exudate |
|---|---|
| Transudate is caused by disturbances of hydrostatic or colloid osmotic pressure and not by inflammation. | An exudate is any fluid that filters from the circulatory system into areas of inflammation. |
| Transudate is extravascular fluid due to an ultrafiltrate of blood plasma. It results from increased fluid pressures or diminished colloid oncotic forces in the plasma. | Exudate is extravascular fluid due to vessel alteration during inflammation due to increased permeability, vascular constriction and then dilation. |
| Transudate is low in protein content and with low specific gravity (< 1.012). | Exudate is high in protein content and high specific gravity (>1.020). |

*Contd...*

*Contd...*

| Transudate | Exudate |
|---|---|
| It has low nucleated cell counts (less than 1000/microlit) of mononuclear cells: macrophages, lymphocytes and mesothelia cells. | Its composition includes water and the dissolved solutes, it contains plasma proteins, white blood cells, platelets and red blood cells in the case of local vascular damage. |
| Being ultrafiltrate larger molecules such as proteins and cell debris are absent. | Cell debris is present. |

## PULMONARY TUBERCULOSIS

Radiographic findings in pulmonary tuberculosis are divided into two forms. Primary tuberculosis represents the initial infection with mycobacterium bacilli in an unsensitized host. Post primary tuberculosis is caused by reactivation of latent foci infection implanted during primary tuberculosis.

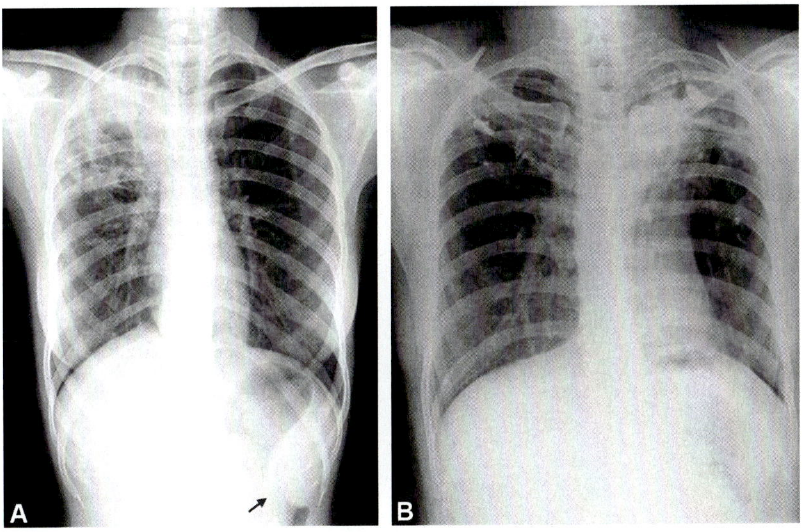

**Figs 2.9A and B:** (A) Chest X-ray non-homogeneous fibro patchy nodular lesions involving the entire right upper lobe with volume loss with resultant pulling up of right hilum. These are features of active lesion and also shows enlarged spleen (arrow); (B) Another case shows multiple calcified lesions are seen in both lungs essentially in the upper lobes. Marked fibrosis in left upper zone as a result mediastinum is pulled to the left and left hilum is pulled up. There is also fibrosis in right upper zone with the right hilum pulled up

Primary tuberculosis manifest as a homogeneous area of parenchymal consolidation typically in the mid or lower zone, associated mediastinal lymphadenopathy is seen. The parenchymal lesion resolves by calcification and is referred as Ghon's focus.

Tuberculoma appear as mass like opacities, usually less than 3 cm in size and located predominantly in the upper lobes.

Postprimary tuberculosis occurs as a result of reactivation of dormant tubercular bacilli due to immunosuppression, malnutrition or old age. It occurs exclusively in the adults. Reactivation usually occurs in the secondary foci in the apical and posterior segments of the upper lobes or superior segments of lower lobes. Characteristic features are predilection for the upper lobes with infiltrates, (Figs 2.9A and B) generally absence of lymphadenopathy and propensity for cavitations, areas of bronchiectasis occur as a complication. Infiltration resolves by fibrosis and calcification.

## MILIARY TUBERCULOSIS

Miliary tuberculosis results from hematogenous or bronchogenic spread from the primary focus. It is seen commonly in the elderly and children below 2 years of age and in immunocompromised patients.

Radiological features on chest X-ray are multiple, well-defined, 2-5 mm miliary mottling of roughly the same size, diffusely and evenly distributed throughout the lung fields with slight lower lobe predominance (Figs 2.10 and 2.11).

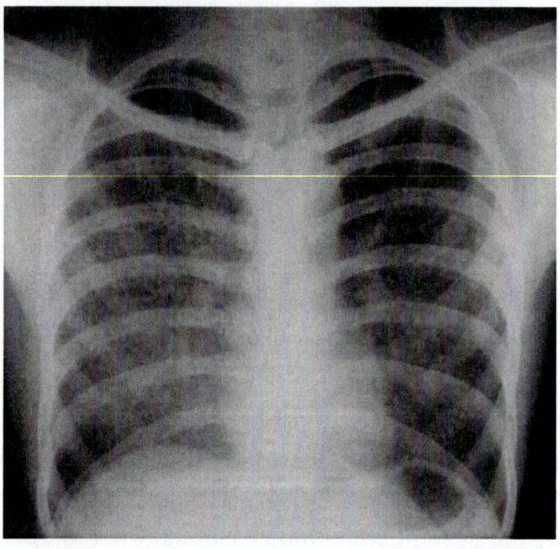

Fig. 2.10: There are multiple small rounded densities of roughly the same size scattered through both lungs. This pattern of small nodules is called 'miliary'. No hila or mediastinal adenopathy can be seen

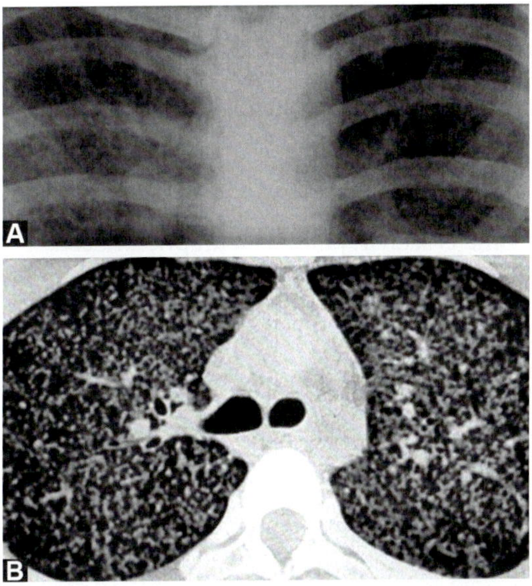

Figs 2.11A and B: (A) Enlarged view of Fig. 2.10; (B) CT scan of the same patient which shows findings same as the X-ray. However, on CT the miliary nodules are discrete, roughly the same size scattered through both lungs

High resolution CT is more sensitive in detection of these nodules. These nodules may enlarge and coalesce to form areas of consolidation if untreated. Ground glass opacities are second most common finding in miliary tuberculosis

The differential includes sarcoidosis, metastases or silicosis, and occupational lung disease from exposure to silica dust.

## PNEUMOCONIOSIS

It comprises group of diffuse lung diseases due to inhalation of small inorganic dust particles. The dust particles ingested by alveolar macrophages results in their breakdown with release of enzymes which produce fibrogenic response. It takes 10-20 years of exposure before appreciated on X-ray. Pneumoconiosis has a progressive course despite cessation to dust exposure. On imaging multiple diffuse small nodular rounded opacities 1-10 mm in size are seen (Figs 2.12 and 2.13), may have ground-glass appearance and may occasionally calcify. Lymph node enlargement is common. Examples are silicosis, asbestosis and coal worker's pneumoconiosis.

X-ray shows multiple nodular shadows in the upper and mid zones. Areas of bizarre shaped calcifications are noted involving pleura particularly diaphragmatic pleura suggest asbestosis.

HRCT in addition to the nodular opacities also demonstrates areas of parenchymal fibrosis and septal lines. Egg shell calcification is noted involving hilar lymph nodes.

Complication include pulmonary hypertension and cor pulmonale, Caplan's syndrome is seen in patients with pneumoconiosis and rheumatoid arthritis.

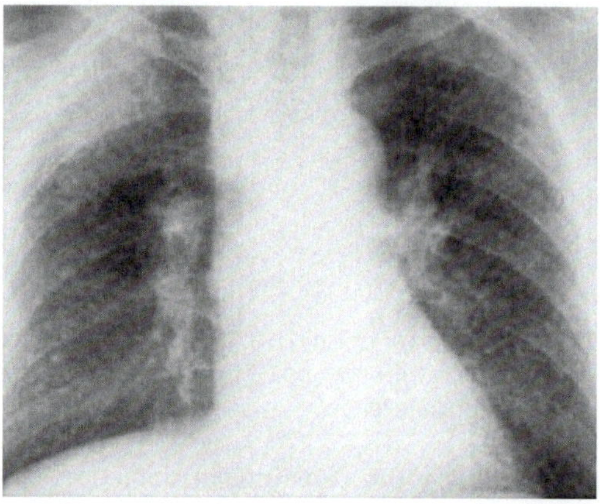

**Fig. 2.12:** Chest X-ray shows multiple small nodular dense opacities are seen in both lungs with hilar adenopathy in an asbestos-cement factory worker (occupational lung disease)

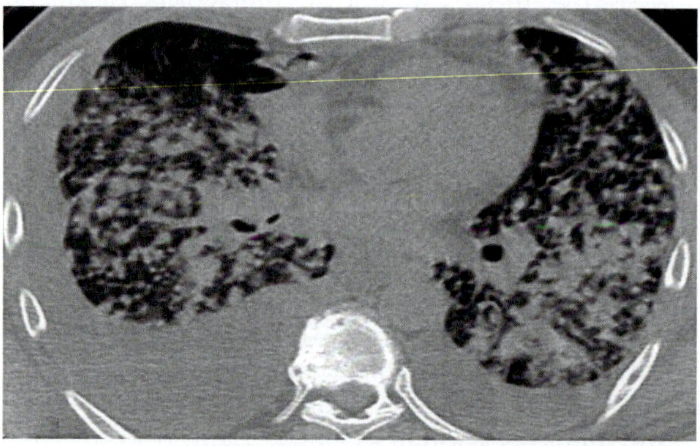

**Fig. 2.13:** CT chest shows multiple small nodular dense opacities are seen in both lungs with bilateral effusion and hilar adenopathy in a case of pneumoconiosis

## PNEUMOTHORAX

Presence of the air within the pleural cavity is termed as the pneumothorax. Air enters into the pleural cavity through the defect in pleural layers either spontaneously or due to trauma. Spontaneous pneumothorax when seen in healthy individuals without any precipitating event is known as primary spontaneous pneumothorax in contrast to the secondary spontaneous pneumothorax which is seen in the setting of a predisposing lung disease like chronic obstructive pulmonary disease (COPD). Traumatic pneumothorax is more common and is seen in patients undergoing mechanical ventilation. Traumatic pneumothorax occurs due to blunt or penetrating chest trauma.

On erect X-ray PA view chest shows presence of radiolucent pleural space devoid of vascular markings and seen separating visceral pleura from chest wall (Fig. 2.14). Lung apex is seen retracted towards the hilum with partial collapse of underlying lung.

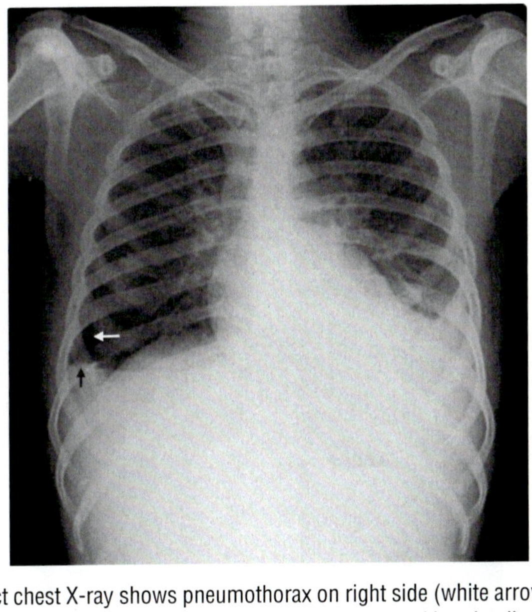

Fig. 2.14: Erect chest X-ray shows pneumothorax on right side (white arrow) at the inferior end of pneumothorax is a small air fluid level (black arrow) making the diagnosis as hydropneumothorax

## Tension Pneumothorax

Tension pneumothorax is pneumothorax with air under pressure in the pleural space. This condition is most common following trauma or mechanical ventilation resulting in one way valve, allowing air to enter the pleural space and preventing the air from escaping naturally. This condition can rapidly progress to respiratory insufficiency, cardiovascular collapse and life-threatening if goes unrecognized and untreated. Favorable patient outcome requires urgent diagnosis and immediate management by needle decompression of the pleural space.

It is a clinical emergency characterized by tachypnea, tachycardia, decreased or absent breath sounds, cyanosis and hypotension.

On chest X-ray the air under pressure in the pleural space results in hyperlucent (black) hemithorax devoid of vascular markings, collapse of lung on the side of pneumothorax and the diaphragm is depressed. The mediastinum is pushed to the contralateral side (Fig. 2.15), arrows show the medial margin of the right pleura which is actually herniating into the left hemithorax.

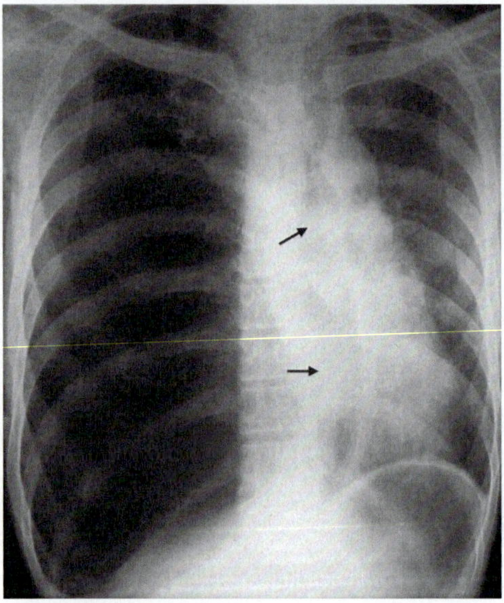

Fig. 2.15: Chest X-ray shows a hyperlucent lung on right side with inversion of right dome of diaphragm and mediastinal shift to opposite side (arrows) herniating into the left hemithorax

Treatment is by immediate placement of the wide bore needle in the second intercostal space in the midclavicular line and nasal oxygen is given and intercostal drainage (ICD) insertion is done patient is stabilized. Ventilatory support with intermittent positive pressure ventilation (IPPV) is given in severe cases.

### Open Pneumothorax

Open pneumothorax is where the pleural cavity communicates with the external environment. It is generally due to penetrating trauma. It presents with breathlessness, tachypnea, hyper-resonant note, absent or decreased breath sounds.

Complications of open pneumothorax are:

a. Hydropneumothorax, pyopneumothorax, hemopneumothorax
b. Tension pneumothorax
c. Pneumomediastinum.

Chest X-ray shows unilateral hyperlucency on the affected side with absence of lung markings and collapsed lung margins with air fluid level. Treatment is by insertion of an intercostal drainage (ICD) and treating the cause.

## ASPERGILLOMA/FUNGAL BALL

*Aspergillus* is a common fungus and grows on dead leaves, stored grain, bird droppings, compost piles and decaying vegetation.

Aspergillomas also known as fungal ball are formed when the *aspergillus* grows in a clump in a cavity. It is seen in the lung cavities commonly. Most patients with pulmonary aspergillosis have either an underlying pre-existing chronic lung disease or impaired immunity. Examples of pre-existing chronic lung disease include tuberculosis, bronchiectasis, sarcoidosis, lung abscess, lung cancer, and cystic fibrosis. Fungal ball can also be seen in the brain, kidney, or other organs.

Patients are usually asymptomatic. Few patients present with chest pain, cough, fever, and hemoptysis.

On chest X-ray the characteristic appearance of round or oval soft-tissue opacity mass. Often, an adjacent crescent-shaped air space (i.e. the air-crescent sign) separates the fungal ball from the cavity wall. The fungal ball is usually mobile and moves when the patient changes position (Figs 2.16A and B).

On CT scan the fungal ball is seen as a mass of soft-tissue attenuation within a pulmonary cavity. An anterior air crescent is visible if the patient is supine. In the prone position; the fungal ball falls to the dependent portion of the cavity (Figs 2.17A and B).

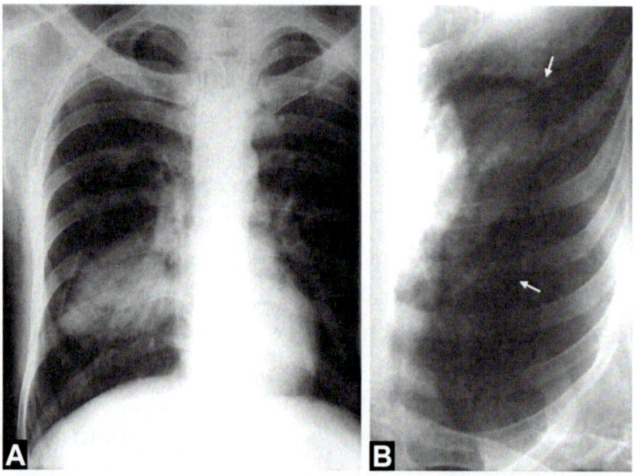

**Figs 2.16A and B:** 43-year-old male presented with cough fever and weight loss with loss of appetite since two months: (A) Chest X-ray PA view, demonstrates a well-defined cavity in right lower zone with fairly well-demarcated opacity seen in it. On lateral projection it was to be located in superior segment of right lower lung; (B) On chest radiograph taken in trendelenburg (head low) position, opacity within the cavity has moved superiorly. These are typical features of a fungal ball

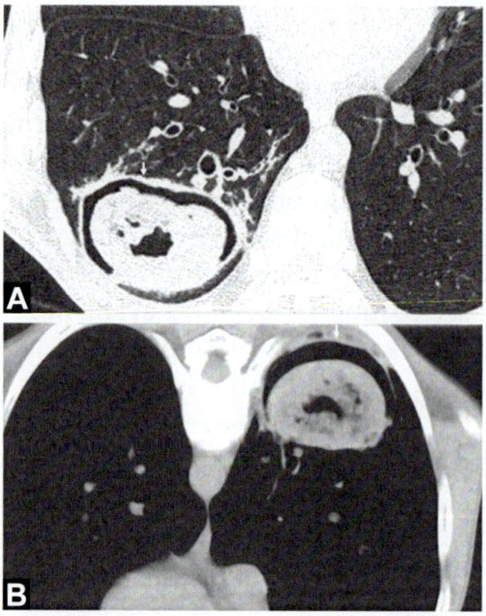

**Figs 2.17A and B:** CT chest showed a thick-walled cavity in the right lower lobe with a fungal ball inside the cavity: (A) Fungal ball moved to the dependent position; (B) When CT chest was performed in prone position. This fungal ball was caused by *Candida albicans* as confirmed by transbronchial biopsy

## HYDATID CYST

Hydatid disease is infestation by Echinococcus granulosus (parasitic tapeworm).

*Life cycle:* Echinococcus granulosus tapeworm lives in the intestine of the dog (definitive host). The dog excretes the eggs in the feces which when swallowed by the intermediate hosts-humans, sheep, cattle, goats, the embryos are released from the egg into the duodenum and pass through the mucosa to the liver through the portal venous system. Most of the embryos remain trapped in the liver, although may reach lungs, kidneys, spleen, CNS and bone.

In the liver, the right lobe is more commonly involved. Surviving embryo develops into a slow growing cyst. The cyst wall consists of an external membrane that is approximately 1 mm thick called ectocyst which may calcify. Host forms a dense connective tissue capsule around the cyst termed as pericyst (Figs 2.18 and 2.19). The inner germinal layer or the endocyst gives rise to brood capsules that enlarge to form protoscolises. The brood capsules may separate from the wall and form fine sediment called hydatid sand. When hydatid cysts within the organ of a herbivore are eaten, the scolioses attach to the intestine and grow to adult tapeworm, thus completing life cycle.

USG features can be similar to a simple cysts with acoustic enhancement, it may contain some hydatid sand, daughter cysts may be present. The cyst may become densely calcified.

Treatment is by surgery. Percutaneous drainage of cyst under imaging guidance can be done.

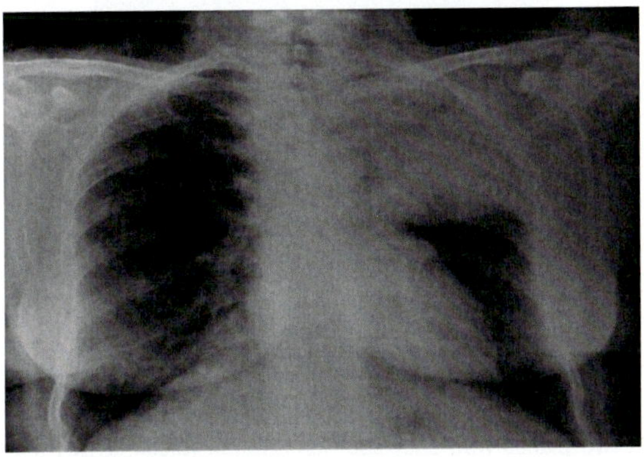

**Fig. 2.18:** X-ray PA view chest shows a 5 × 6 cm oval to circular lesion located in the apex of the left lung likely to be a cyst

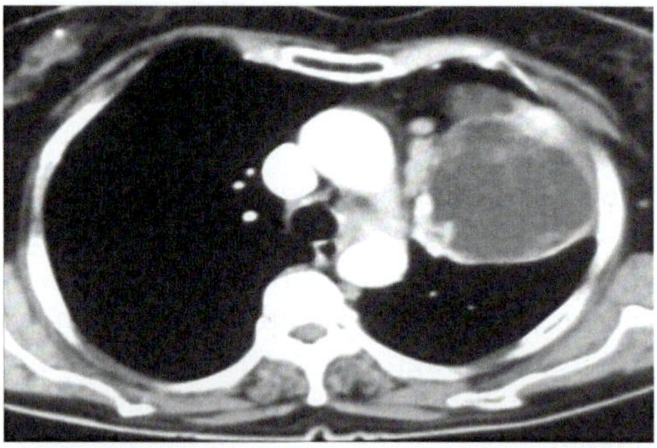

**Fig. 2.19:** CT scan chest of same case as in Figure 2.18 at the level of aortic arch confirms a round cystic lesion in the left lung upper lobe with enhancement of the wall, another small cystic lesion is lying anterior to this. It was diagnosed as hydatid cysts

## FLAIL CHEST

A critical condition following major blunt chest trauma in which two or more contiguous ribs are fractured at two or more places, a segment of the thoracic cage is separated from the rest of the chest (flail segment), as a result a part of the chest wall moves freely in the opposite direction as to the rest of the chest (Fig. 2.20). The related complications are pneumothorax, pleural effusion, pulmonary laceration and contusion.

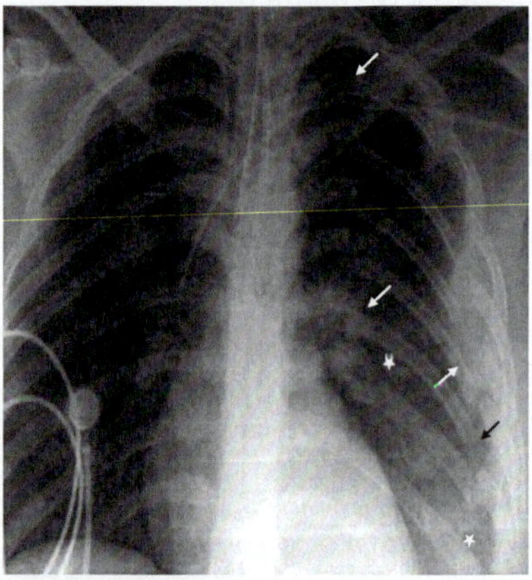

**Fig. 2.20:** Anteroposterior view of chest shows 3rd to 8th rib fractures (white arrows) on left side, each at two places with encysted hemothorax (black arrow) and lung contusion (extends between the asterisks) with diaphragm pushed down and mediastinal shift to the right side

Treatment includes alteration of position to make the patient most comfortable and provide relief of pain, good analgesia with intercostal block and positive pressure ventilation. Surgical fixation is usually not required.

## KARTAGENER'S SYNDROME

Kartagener syndrome is situs inversus (reversal of the internal organs) accompanied by bronchiectasis and chronic sinusitis. Most cases are observed before the age of 15 years. Etiology is unknown with autosomal recessive inheritance.

Symptoms and sign are dyspnea, productive cough, recurrent respiratory infection, cold, pneumonia, rheumatoid arthritis, anosmia and clubbing of fingers (Figs 2.21A to F).

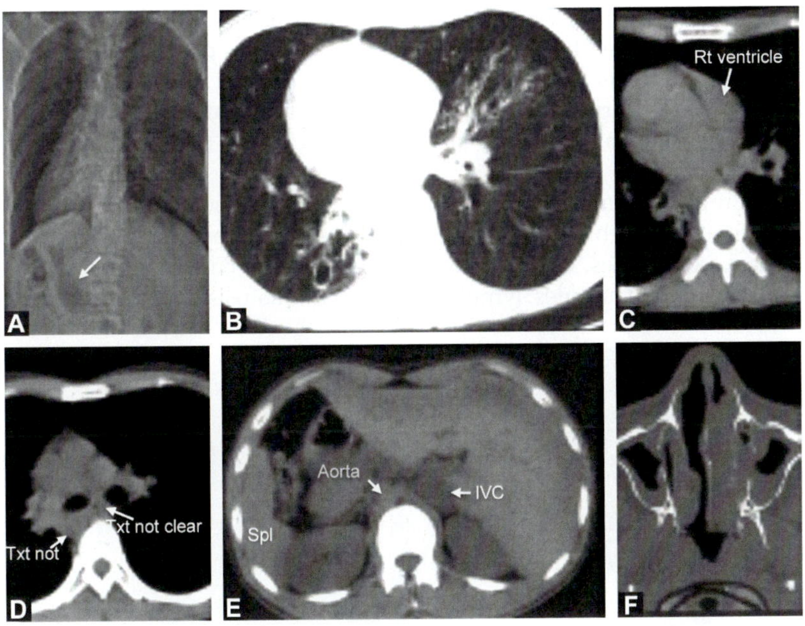


**Figs 2.21A to F:** (A) X-ray shows situs inversus with heart and stomach (arrow) on the right side; (B) Axial CT chest shows bronchiectasis, dextrocardia wirh morphologic right ventricle on the left and the left ventricle on the right; (C to E) Plain axial CT at the level of renals shows liver and IVC on the left and the spleen and aorta on the right; (F) Axial CT PNS shows chronic sinusitis in an individual with Kartagener syndrome

## TUMORS OF THE LUNG

Lung tumors are classified as:

1. Primary
   a. Benign-Pulmonary hamartoma
   b. Malignant-Carcinoma of bronchus, alveolar cell carcinoma, lymphoma and carcinoid
2. Metastases

   Most common fatal malignancy in the adult males is carcinoma of the bronchus. Carcinoma bronchus is of four types-squamous cell carcinoma, adenocarcinoma, small cell carcinoma and large cell carcinoma. On chest X-ray it presents as central or peripherally situated mass (Figs 2.22 and 2.23). Features suggesting malignancy are nodular mass with irregular, spiculated margins; cavitating mass lesion with thick irregular or nodular walls. It may be associated with hilar enlargement or segmental or lobar collapse of the lung.

   Carcinoma of the apex of the lung is termed as pancoast's tumor or superior sulcus tumor. It manifests with distinct clinical features of Horner's syndrome due to involvement of brachial plexus.

   CT is indicated for the staging of carcinoma lung and detecting metastasis.

   Lung is the most common site for metastatic disease. Most common primaries are breast, gastrointestinal tract, kidney, testes, head and neck, and bones. On imaging it shows various patterns like multiple parenchymal nodules, lymphangitis carcinomatosis or pleural effusion.

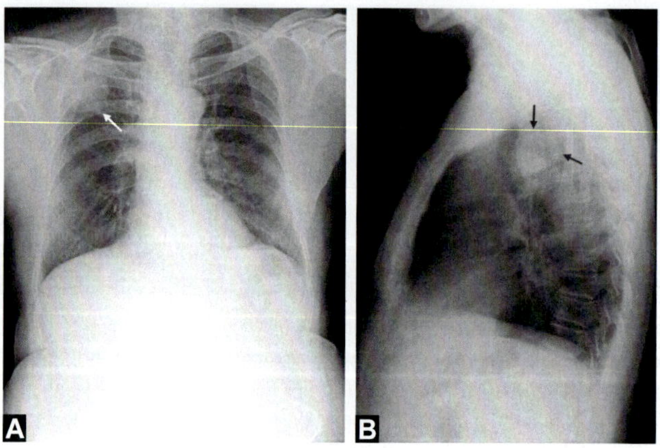


**Figs 2.22A and B:** (A) Chest X-ray PA; (B) Lateral views show a mass lesion in right upper lobe (arrow) in a 70-year-old male, likely bronchogenic carcinoma

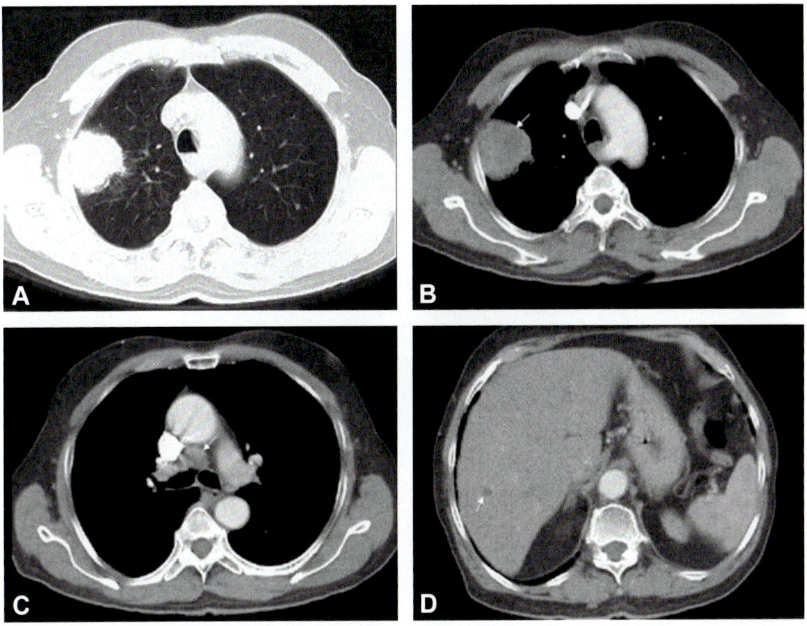


**Figs 2.23A to D:** CT of the case in Fig. 2.22 confirms the diagnosis: (A and B) Show ill-defined rounded opacity abutting the chest wall wit radiating strand seen in right upper lobe with minimal necrosis within seen in mediastinal window; (C) Mediastinal window shows aortopulmonary lymph node (arrow); (D) A small round hypodense metastases is seen in the right lobe of liver

## PANCOAST TUMOR

Carcinoma of the apex of the lung is termed as pancoast tumor or superior sulcus tumor (Figs 2.24 and 2.25) that may involves the brachial plexus and sympathetic ganglion of the lower neck and upper mediastinum Bronchogenic carcinoma or metastatic lesion are the most common causes of pancoast tumors, other causes are lymphoma, mesothelioma, and multiple myeloma.

Pancoast syndrome is a clinical triad of: (1) Horner's syndrome—ptosis, miosis, anhidrosis, and enophthalmos, (2) Ipsilateral arm pain, (3) Wasting of the hand muscles. The pancoast tumors are best depicted.

The pancoast tumors are best depicted on the coronal and sagittal MR images (Fig. 2.26).

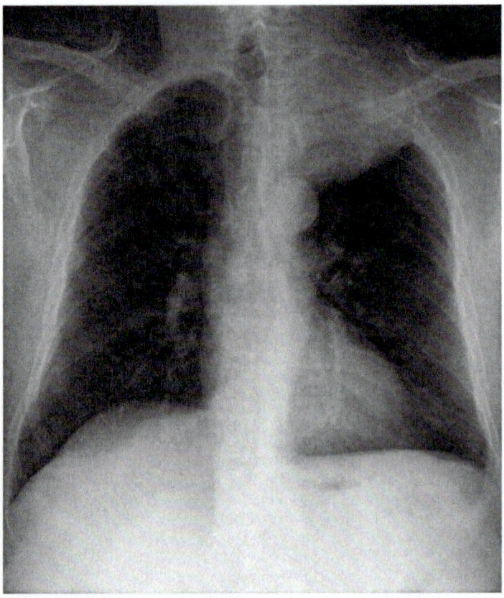

Fig. 2.24: Chest X-ray shows a mass lesion occupying left apex with trachea pushed to the right

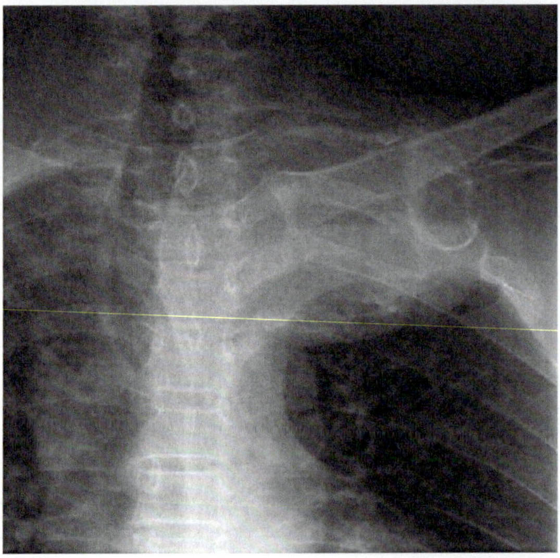

Fig. 2.25: Penetrated view chest in addition to mass in the left apex shows destruction of 1st and 2nd ribs on the left

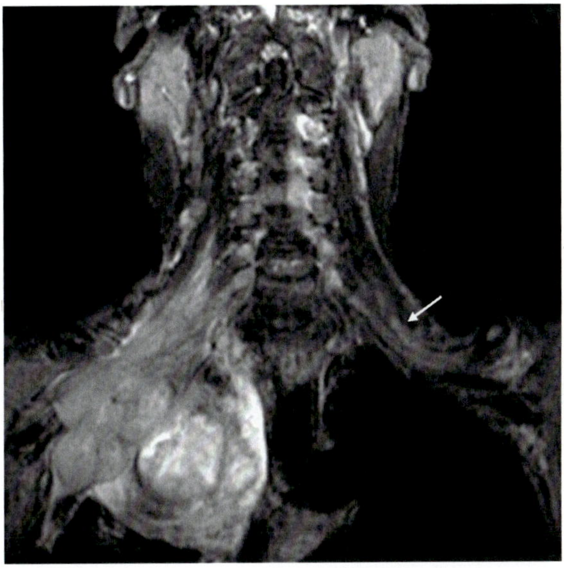

Fig. 2.26: In an another case MRI shows a large heterogenous lesion is seen in the apex of right lung involving the ribs, brachial plexus and adjacent soft tissues. Brachial plexus is normal on left side (arrow)

## SOLITARY PULMONARY NODULE OR COIN LESION

Solitary pulmonary nodule (SPN) refers to a single, focal, round or ovoid lesion of the lung parenchyma measuring up to 3 cm in the diameter detected on chest X-ray without any associated adenopathy, atelectasis or consolidation (Fig. 2.27). If the size is more than 3 cm it is referred as mass lesion.

Differential diagnosis of SPN

1. Infections
   a. Granulomatous lesions—Tuberculoma, histoplasmosis
   b. Round pneumonia
   c. Lung abscess
   d. Hydatid cyst
2. Congenital—Pulmonary sequestration
3. Neoplasms
   a. Benign—Hamartoma and bronchogenic cyst
   b. Malignant—Bronchogenic carcinoma, metastasis and lymphoma
4. Vascular—Hematoma and infarct.

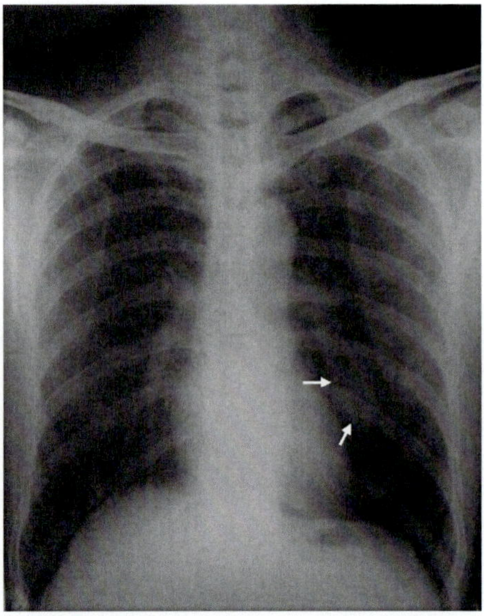

Fig. 2.27: Chest X-ray shows solitary pulmonary nodule or coin lesion (arrows) in left lung field in paracardiac location

## HAMARTOMA

Hamartoma is a benign lesion with aberrant differentiation producing a mass of disorganized but mature specialized cells or tissue indigenous to a particular site leading to overgrowth of tissues.

Examples are hemangiomas, lymphangiomas and A-V malformation.

Pulmonary hamartoma is a tumor which consists of an abnormal arrangement of the tissues normally found in the organ concerned. They most often present as a solitary pulmonary nodule (SPN) in an asymptomatic adult.

Chest radiograph shows a peripherally situated, well circumscribed SPN of varying size. They do not cavitate and show characteristic "popcorn calcification".

CT scan is diagnostic in pulmonary hamartoma.

## MULTIPLE PULMONARY NODULES

Multiple Pulmonary nodules in lung (Figs 2.28A and B), the differential diagnosis includes:

1. Infections
   a. Granulomas—Tuberculomas, histoplasmosis or fungal granulomas
   b. Round pneumonias
   c. Septic emboli
   d. Lung abscess
   e. Hydatid cyst
2. Inflammatory conditions
   a. Rheumatoid arthritis
   b. Caplan's syndrome
   c. Wegener's granulomatosis
   d. Sarcoidosis
3. Neoplasms
   a. Benign—Hamartoma, laryngeal papillomatosis.
   b. Malignant—Metastatic carcinoma, sarcoma, lymphoma.
4. Others are progressive massive fibrosis and hematomas

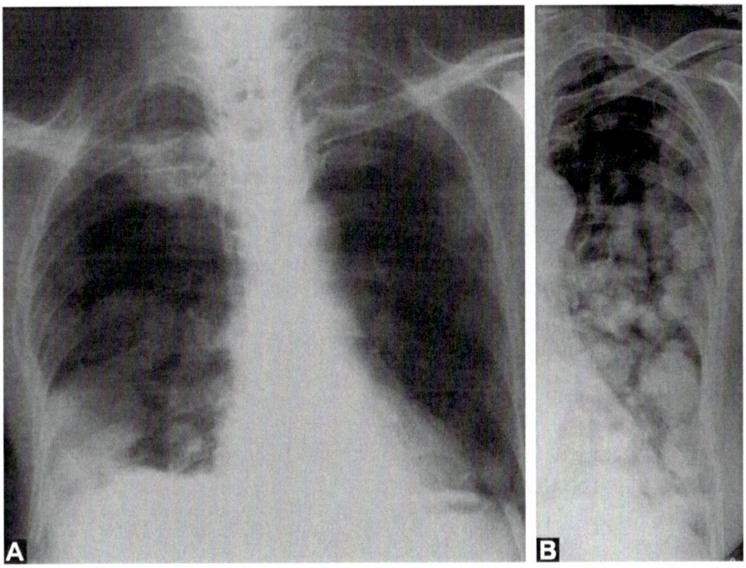


**Figs 2.28A and B:** Two different cases on chest X-ray lung fields show multiple metastases of different sizes involving all lobes of both lungs

CHAPTER 3

# Heart

**Chapter Outline**

- Pericardial Effusion
- Tetralogy of Fallot
- Mitral Stenosis
- Ventricular Septal Defect
- Atrial Septal Defect

## PERICARDIAL EFFUSION

Pericardial effusion is accumulation of fluid in the pericardial space. A normal pericardial sac contains about 30 ml of pericardial fluid. Pericardial effusion with enough pressure to adversely affect heart function is called cardiac tamponade.

Causes of pericardial effusion are:

a. Idiopathic
b. Inflammatory
    i. Postmyocardial infarction (Dressler's syndrome)
    ii. Connective tissue disorders
c. Infectious
    i. Viral
    ii. Bacterial
    iii. Tubercular
d. Postsurgical/trauma
e. Radiotherapy
f. Malignancy
    i. Primary: e.g. pericardial mesothelioma
    ii. Metastatic

g. Metabolic
i. Hypothyroidism

Patient presents with chest pain, breathlessness, dyspnea on exertion. A small effusion may be asymptomatic.

### On Chest X-ray

a. A very small pericardial effusion may not be evident on plain film.
b. Heart appears as a globular enlargement giving a "water bottle" configuration (Fig. 3.1).
c. Lateral chest X-ray may show an "Oreo Cookie Sign": a vertical lucent line directly behind sternum (epicardial fat), behind this a vertical opaque line (pericardial fluid) and behind this a vertical lucent line (pericardial fat).
d. Widening of the subcarinal angle without other evidence of left atrial enlargement may be an indirect clue.

2D ECHO is diagnostic as it shows separation of epicardial and pericardial echoes by fluid. Volume of fluid can be estimated. It can be used as a therapeutic modality to aspirate the pericardial fluid.

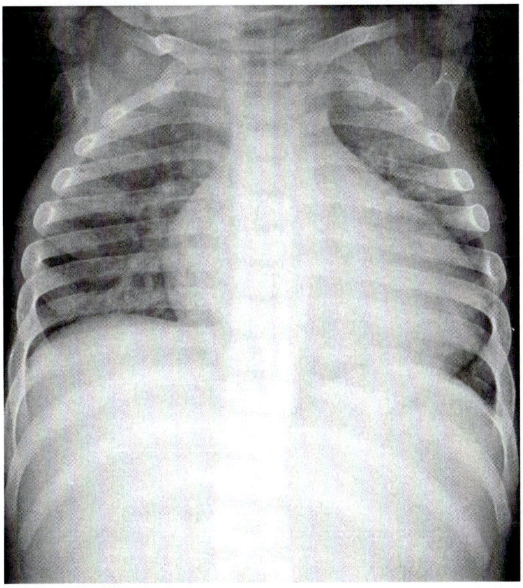

Fig. 3.1: Heart appears as a globular enlargement giving a water bottle configuration

## TETRALOGY OF FALLOT

Tetralogy of Fallot is the most common cyanotic heart disease. Morphologic abnormalities of tetralogy of Fallot are as follows:

i. Right ventricular outflow tract obstruction
ii. Ventricular septal defect
iii. Right ventricular hypertrophy
iv. Over-riding of aorta.

On chest X-ray the right ventricular hypertrophy is seen as elevated left ventricle. Combined with a small or absent main pulmonary artery segment, the heart shows the classic boot-shaped appearance (Fig. 3.2). Vascularity of the pulmonary artery is reduced. A right-sided arch is present in 25% of cases.

Echocardiography is the primary imaging method in suspected cases. Echocardiography should be used to confirm radiographic findings that are suggestive of tetralogy of Fallot. Intracardiac anomalies, including pulmonary infundibular and valvular stenosis and the position of the aortic root over-riding and the ventricular septal defect are identified.

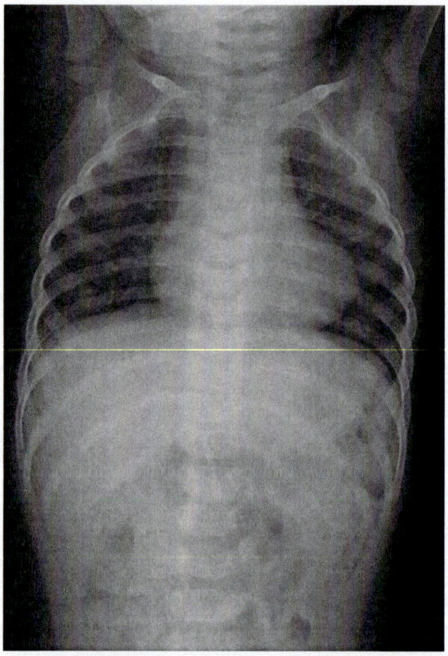

**Fig. 3.2:** Chest X-ray of a one-year-old child shows a boot-shaped heart produced by elevated left ventricle combined with a small or absent main pulmonary artery segment and vascularity of the pulmonary artery is reduced

CT is useful for the evaluation of surgical complications such as infection or pseudoaneurysm formation. Also to identify airway compression that is caused by a large ascending aorta that is associated with tetralogy of Fallot and MRI can be used to identify the morphologic abnormalities.

Cardiac catheterization and angiography is often required in addition to echocardiography because precise assessment of anatomy is essential in surgical planning.

## MITRAL STENOSIS

Mitral stenosis (MS) results in the reduction of blood flow across the mitral valve due to fusion of leaflet commissures. The most common cause of MS is rheumatic fever. Chest radiograph provides useful information about the cardiac size, pulmonary vasculature, arterial and venous hypertension and secondary changes in the lung. Cardiac size may be normal.

The hallmark of MS is selective mild-to-moderate left atrial (LA) enlargement which results in straightening of the left heart border to a large bulge immediately below the left main bronchus. Secondary signs of LA enlargement are upward displacement of left main bronchus resulting in widening of carinal angle (Figs 3.3A and B) and deviation of the middle third of descending thoracic aorta to the left (Bedford sign).

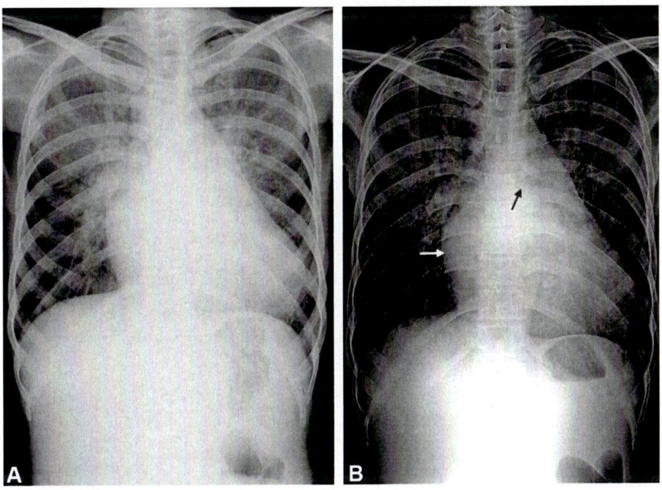


**Figs 3.3A and B:** Chest X-ray in mitral stenosis. Double density due to enlarged left atrium (white arrow) is seen and there is increased carinal angle (black arrow). Normal carinal angle is 40-65$^0$. The left heart border is straightened. There is prominence of upper lobe vessels in the lungs as appreciated by increased density in upper lobes

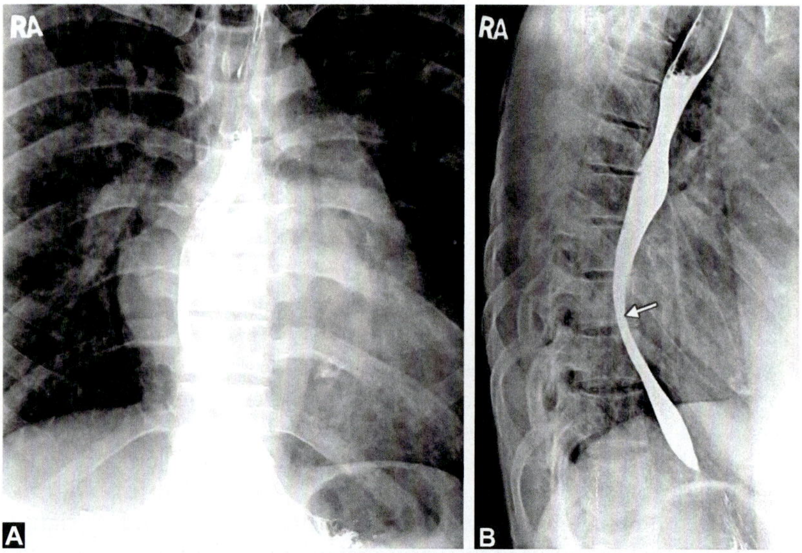


**Figs 3.4A and B:** C-shaped extrinsic impression on the esophagus pushing it to the right (A) and (B) posteriorly (arrow) due to enlarged left atrium

Calcification of mitral valve if seen suggest rheumatic etiology. Hemodynamic changes in the pulmonary circulation are sensitive indicators of the severity of the disease displayed as prominence of upper lobe vessels, diminution of lower lobe vessels (Figs 3.3A and B), Kerley B lines and pleural effusion suggests pulmonary venous hypertension.

Enlargement of the main and branch pulmonary arteries indicate pulmonary arterial hypertension. Double right heart border is due to enlargement of left atrium. Hemosiderosis and ossific pulmonary nodules are noted in chronic long standing cases. Esophagus is pushed posteriorly and to the right (Figs 3.4A and B) due to enlarged left atrium.

2D echocardiography identifies and quantifies the severity of stenotic valve lesion and valve morphology. Doppler helps to assess the trans-stenotic pressure gradient.

## Ventricular Septal Defect

Ventricular septal defect (VSD) is a left to right shunt (L to R shunt) and is most common cyanotic heart disease in children. During embryological development single ventricular chamber divides into two by fusion of membranous portion of ventricular septum with endocardial cushions and bulbous cordis. VSD is classified based on the derangement in the development of one of these structures:

i. Membranous VSD
ii. Supracristal or Conal VSD
iii. Muscular VSD
iv. Atrioventricular or Endocardial cushion type.

It usually manifests after birth when pulmonary pressure decreases and systemic arterial pressure increases with development of L to R shunt.

Chest X-ray shows variable appearance depending on the size of the defect. It shows cardiomegaly with enlargement of left atrium, left ventricle and right ventricle. Pulmonary artery segment appears enlarged with increased pulmonary vascularity. 2D ECHO helps to identify and classify the VSD. Pressure gradient across the defect can be determined.

Cross-sectional imaging CT and MRI are helpful in complicated cases to detect associated vascular anomalies and preoperative planning.

## ATRIAL SEPTAL DEFECT

Atrial septal defect (ASD) is the most common congenital heart disease diagnosed in adults. It is classified into four types:

i. *Ostium secundum ASD:* Exaggerated resorptive process of septum primum
ii. *Ostium primum ASD:* Defect in atrioventricular endocardial cushion
iii. Sinus venosus defect in superior inlet portion of the atrial septum
iv. Coronary sinus defect due to absence of normal coronary sinus.

Hemodynamic changes occur after birth due to increase in physiological pressure of left atrium (LA) with flow of blood from left side of heart to right side of heart, i.e. from LA to right atrium (RA) to right ventricle (RV) and is termed as left to right shunt (L-R shunt ), volume overload is well tolerated during childhood. Later right ventricle dilates leading to right heart failure.

Chest X-ray is usually normal if the shunt is small. In cases of large shunt cardiomegaly and increased pulmonary vascularity is seen. High pulmonary flow is seen as pulmonary plethora. Aorta appears small with normal aortic knob (Fig. 3.5). Hilar dance is due to increased pulsations of central pulmonary arteries on fluoroscopy.

2D ECHO is diagnostic and shows paradoxical motion of interventricular septum due to volume overload of RV, interatrial septum is not visualized. Color Doppler study helps to determine presence and direction of blood flow from interatrial septum crossing LA to RA to RV.

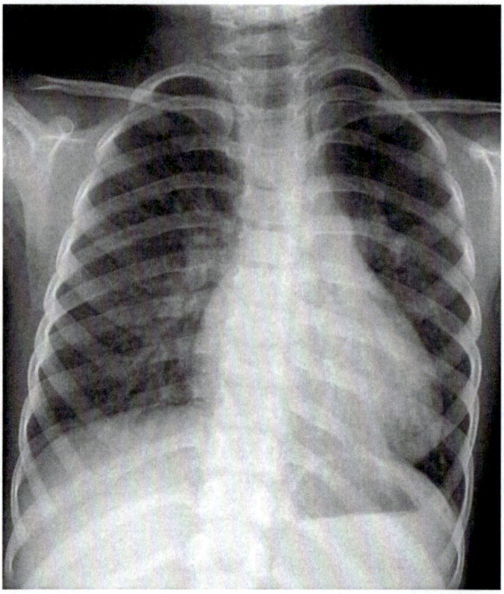

**Fig. 3.5:** ASD—L-R shunt, shows cardiomegaly and pulmonary plethora

CHAPTER 4

# Vascular System

**Chapter Outline**

- Redundant and Tortuous Aorta
- Coarctation of Aorta
- Vascular Calcifications

## REDUNDANT AND TORTUOUS AORTA

Normal configuration of the aorta is maintained due to elasticity of its wall. As age advances there is degenerative change in the elastic fibers of wall, it loses its elasticity and may become redundant and tortuous. Patients usually remain asymptomatic. On chest X-ray it may appear as a widening of the mediastinum. It may mimic aneurysm. However cross sectional imaging confirms the nonaneurysmal tortuous configuration and redundancy of the aorta (Figs 4.1A and B).

### Thoracic Aortic Aneurysm

A true aneurysm is defined as a localized dilatation of the aorta with 50 percent over the normal diameter and includes all three layers of the vessel, intima, media and adventitia. Thoracic aortic aneurysms are less common than aneurysms of the abdominal aorta.

There are two major types of aneurysm morphology: fusiform, and saccular. A pseudoaneurysm or false aneurysm is a collection of blood and connective tissue outside the aortic wall, usually the result of a rupture.

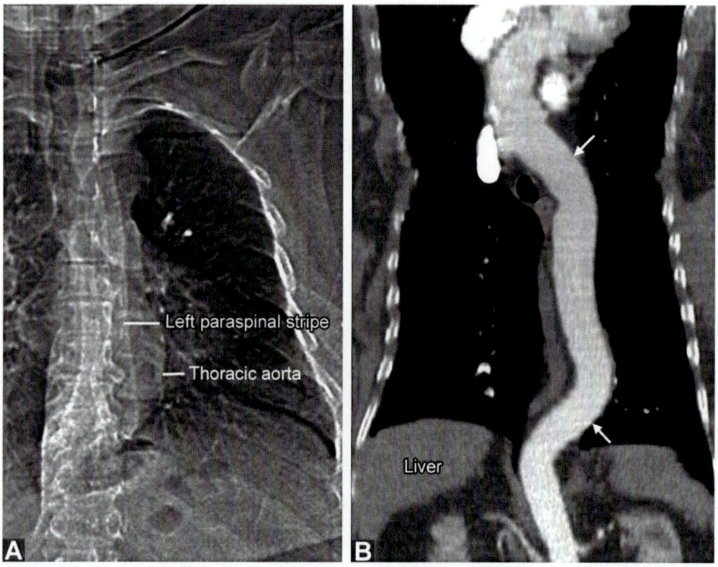


**Figs 4.1A and B:** Scout CT image of chest: (A) Shows prominent descending aorta raising a suspicion of aneurysm. Aortic reconstruction following contrast CT of chest and abdomen; (B) Shows no aneurysm but only tortuous and elongated dilatation of thoracic aorta (arrow)

The incidence of thoracic aortic aneurysm is estimated to be around six cases per lac patient years. Thoracic aneurysms occur most commonly in the sixth and seventh decade of life.

The vast majority of thoracic aneurysms are associated with atherosclerosis male to female ratio is 3:1. Hypertension is an important risk factor, being present in 60 percent of patients.

Asymptomatic aneurysms are incidentally detected on routine X-ray chest. The aortic aneurysm produces mediastinal widening or alter contour of the heart (Figs 4.2A and B).

CT scan with intravenous contrast is a precise diagnostic tool in the evaluation of thoracic aneurysm. The aneurysm size, extend of disease, presence of leakage and coincident pathology (Figs 4.3 and 4.4) is well demonstrated. Magnetic resonance angiography is highly informative with multiplanar image reconstruction and visualization of extraluminal structures but disadvantages being limited availability, increased cost, and lower resolution than traditional contrast angiography.

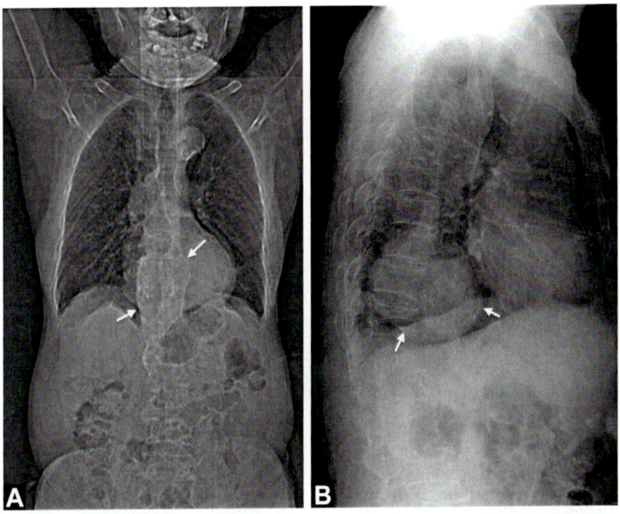

Figs 4.2A and B: X-ray chest on penetrated AP projection: (A) Shows altered contour of distal thoracic aorta (arrow); (B) Lateral view shows the aneurysmal dilatation of distal part of thoracic aorta (arrow)

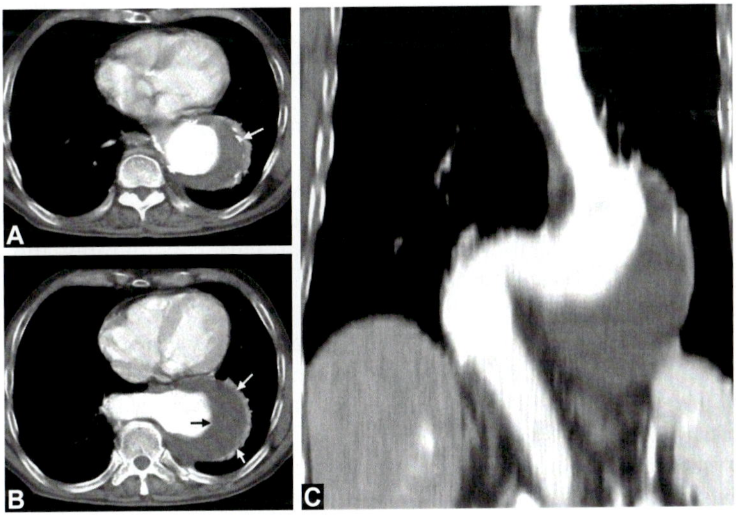

Figs 4.3A to C: Contrast enhanced CT scan (A and B) axial sections; (C) Coronal reformatted image shows a large descending thoracic aorta aneurysm with a large component of intramural thrombus (arrows) which shows no contrast uptake. Calcification is present in the wall abutting the thrombus

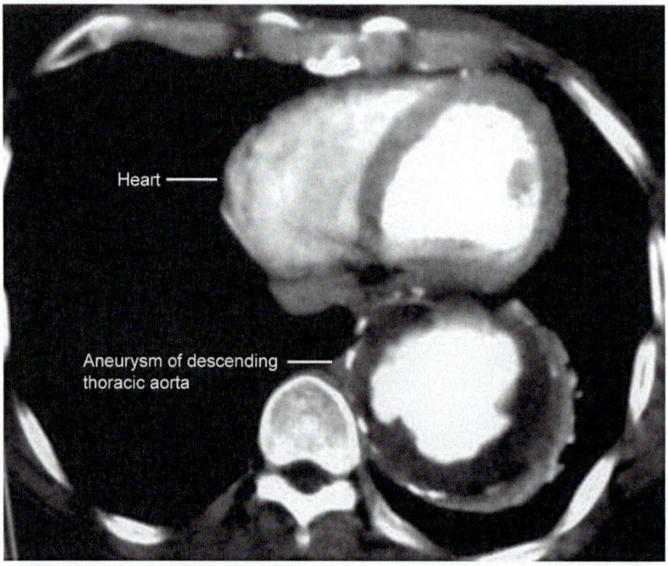


**Fig. 4.4:** In another case contrast CT shows that the lumen of aneurysmal segment is entirely filled with contrast except at periphery, which has hypodense nonenhancing thrombus *in situ*

## COARCTATION OF AORTA

Coarctation of aorta is a congenital aortic narrowing in the region of the isthmus.

There is a characteristic shelf-like narrowing of the aorta which usually occurs just beyond the origin of the left subclavian artery (Figs 4.5A to D). The severity of coarctation or narrowing can vary considerably and it is this severity which determines the age of presentation (Figs 4.5E to G). It is more common in males (M:F = 4.1) and is rare in blacks.

The collateral circulation distal to the coarctation is through the subclavian arteries and its branches like internal mammary artery to intercostals, scapular artery to anterior spinal artery, transverse cervical artery to lateral thoracic artery.

Rib notching (Fig. 4.6) is seen in coarctation of aorta and it usually takes several years to develop. It is due to pressure erosion by the enlarged tortuous collaterals intercostal arteries. It is typically bilateral and is best seen on the inferior aspect of the posterior third of 4th to 9th ribs. It may be unilateral. Chest X-ray showing notching of posterior ribs

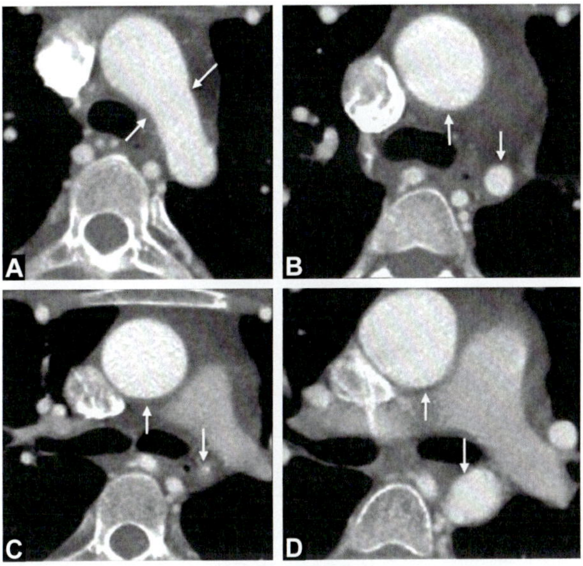


**Figs 4.5A to D:** CT aortic angiography in a case of postductal coarctation of aorta: (A) Aortic arch shows reduction in diameter of descending aorta as compared to ascending (arrow); (B and C) The diameter of ascending aorta (upright arrow) is maintained but that of descending aorta (down pointing arrow) has abruptly reduced; (D) Return of normal caliber of descending aorta

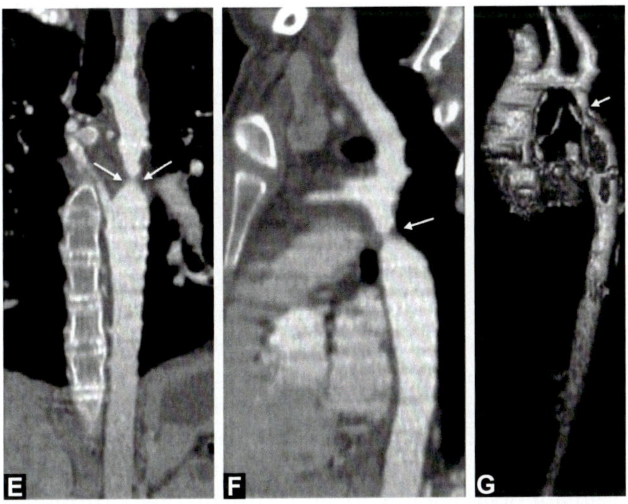


**Figs 4.5E to G:** (E and F) Coronal and sagittal reformatted image shows the actual site of coarctation (arrow); (G) Color coded CT angiogram shows exact location of narrowing (arrow)

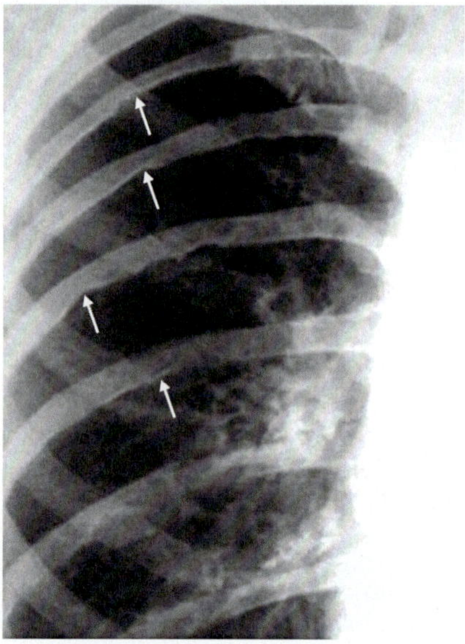

Fig. 4.6: X-ray chest shows rib notching on the inferior aspect of the posterior 4th to 7th ribs (arrow)

bilaterally most prominent along inferior borders is likely a case of aortic coarctation.

## VASCULAR CALCIFICATIONS

For long, passive degeneration is thought to be the cause for vascular calcification. Calcification of blood vessels commonly seen with aging (Figs 4.7 to 4.8), diabetes, atherosclerosis and end stage renal disease (ESRD) is considered a benign finding. However, multislice computed tomography has revolutionized the thought process about the risks of vascular calcification. In coronary arteries, calcification is positively correlated with atherosclerotic plaque with increased risk of myocardial infarction, and plaque instability. Coronary calcification with extent of underlying atherosclerotic disease, contributes to progress of cardiovascular disease.

Vascular calcification found in the media of large arteries, leads to increased stiffening and decreased compliance. Resulting in loss of the cushioning function of these arteries with increased arterial pulse wave velocity and pulse pressure, which leads to impaired arterial distensibility, increased afterload leading to left ventricular hypertrophy, and compromised coronary perfusion.

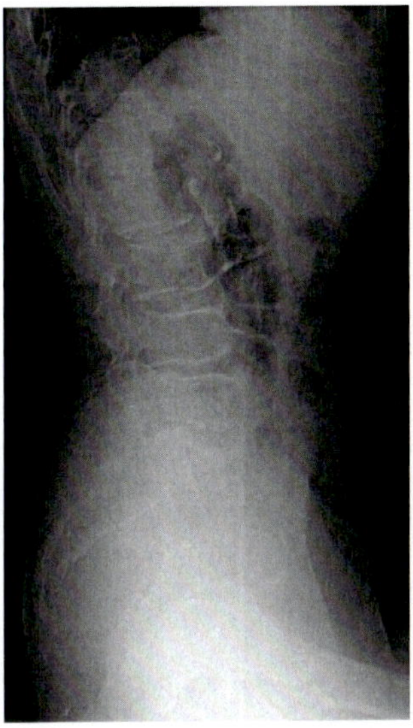

Fig. 4.7: Calcification in the wall of abdominal aorta (arrow)

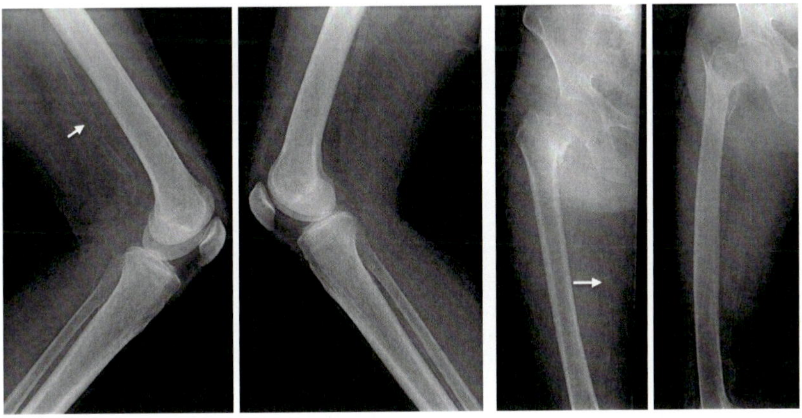

Fig. 4.8: Calcification in the wall popliteal and femoral artery (arrow)

The phlebolithis is the typical finding in venous malformations (Fig. 4.9). The tram track calcification seen in the Struge Weber syndrome is due to calcification in meningeal venous malformation. In venous malformation the pain is usually due to the calcification.

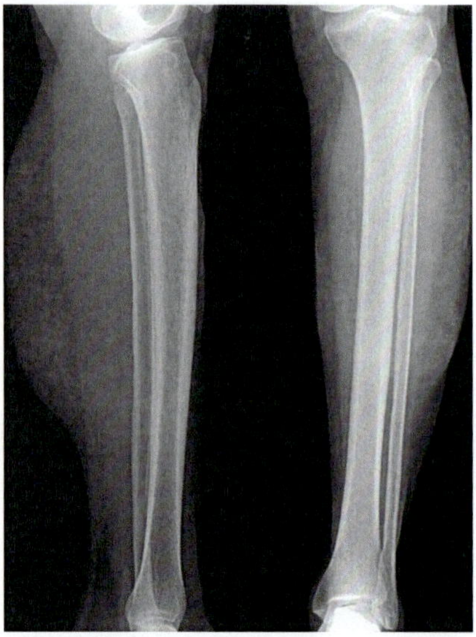

Fig. 4.9: Calcification in venous malformation in the leg

# 5 CHAPTER
# Gastrointestinal Tract and Abdomen

**Chapter Outline**



## TRACHEOESOPHAGEAL FISTULA

The trachea and esophagus develop from the common foregut during early first trimester. Incomplete separation results in esophageal atresia with or without associated tracheo esophageal fistula (T-E fistula).

T-E fistula occurs one in every 3000 to 5000 live births. The neonate usually present later with chocking while feeding, cough, cyanosis, recurrent pneumonia. A naso-gastric tube cannot be passed into the stomach. On X-ray abdomen, it is gasless and may be scaphoid.

### Classification of T-E fistula (Fig. 5.1)

Type A Esophageal atresia without fistula
Type B Esophageal atresia with proximal T-E fistula
Type C Esophageal atresia with distal T-E fistula
Type D Esophageal atresia + proximal and distal T-E fistula
Type E Tracheoesophageal fistula without atresia (H type).

Fifty percent of cases are associated with VACTERL (vertebral, anorectal, cardiac, trachea-esophageal fistula, renal and limb anomalies) syndrome.

Chest radiograph immediately after birth reveals distended proximal esophageal pouch with round distal margin and coiled naso-gastric tube within is diagnostic. The presence of air in the stomach and small bowel indicates esophageal atresia with a distal tracheoesophageal fistula (Fig. 5.1). Absence of air in the stomach eliminates the possibility of a distal fistula.

Use of ionic radiopaque contrast should be avoided. Isotonic nonionic contrast medium should be used in minimal amount under fluoroscopic monitoring.

The best way to demonstrate H-type tracheosophageal fistula is with careful injection of contrast medium via a nasogastric tube.

The side of the aortic arch is identified on imaging because the surgical approach to the mediastinum for repair of esophageal atresia with a distal T-E fistula is from the side opposite the aortic arch.

Antenatal USG feature of polyhydramnios with an absent fluid filled stomach indicates presence of T-E fistula.

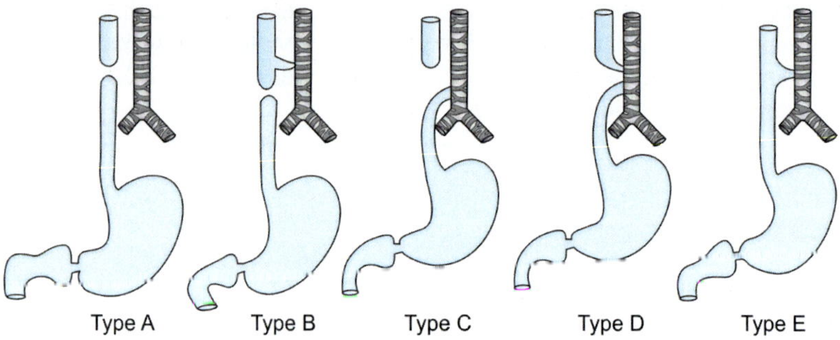


Fig. 5.1: Tracheoesophageal Fistula

## ACHALASIA CARDIA

In achalasia the lower esophageal sphincter does not relax properly leading to impaired emptying of esophagus and gradual dilatation of proximal esophagus.

### Types

Primary achalasia is the most common subtype and results from loss of ganglion cells in the esophageal myenteric plexus.

Secondary achalasia is uncommon and may develop secondary to certain malignancies, diabetes mellitus, and Chagas disease.

Clinical features include dysphagia for solids and liquids, regurgitation of food, pneumonia due to aspiration of food, severe retro sternal chest pain in 30-40% of patients, weight loss and increased risk for esophageal cancer.

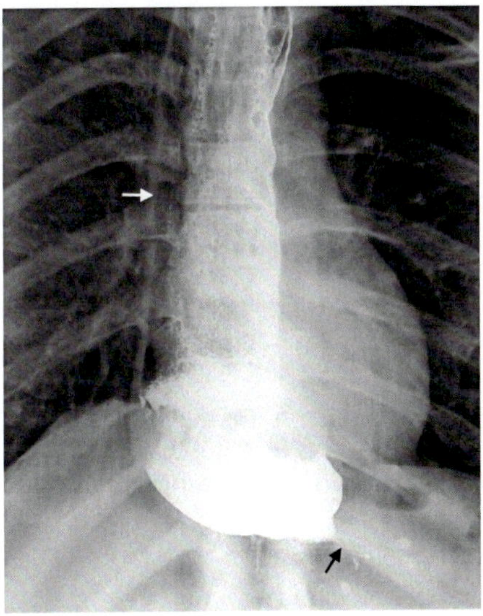

**Fig. 5.2:** Barium swallow shows dilation of the esophagus (white arrow) proximal to the smooth narrowing at lower esophageal sphincter (black arrow)

### Imaging

X-ray chest and abdomen may show air-fluid level in retrocardiac region, non visualization of gastric fundic bubble and aspiration pneumonia.

Barium swallow shows variable degree of dilation of the esophagus with smooth narrowing at lower esophageal sphincter (Figs 5.2 and 5.3). Distal two-third of esophagus may be is aperistaltic.

Upper GI endoscopy shows undigested food particles along with ingested fluid filled esophagus and lower end of esophagus fail to open even after air insufflation.

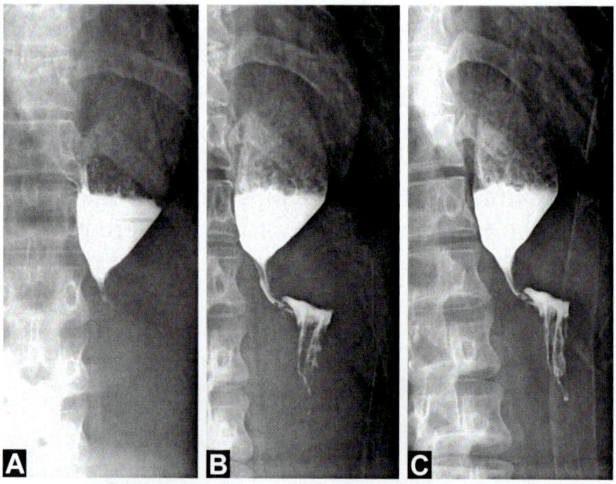

**Figs 5.3A to C:** Another case of achalasia cardia in a relatively early stage shows on barium swallow distended esophagus proximal to the gastroesophageal junction which smoothly tappers to a bird beak appearance

Manometry is gold standard investigation which shows failure of relaxation of lower end of esophagus and pressure at lower end of esophagus may be high.

Endoscopic ultrasound shows thickened muscle layers in the lower part of esophagus.

CT scan demonstrate the structural esophageal abnormalities.

Treatment includes

1. Drugs
    i. Calcium channel blockers
    ii. Anticholinergic agents
    iii. Nitrates and
    iv. Botox injections
2. Endoscopic dilatation
3. Surgical treatment is by Heller's myotomy

## ESOPHAGEAL WEBS

Esophageal webs is a shelf-like infolding of the mucosa protrude into the lumen from the anterior wall of the cervical or thoracic esophagus. They may be semicircular or may form a complete ring (Figs 5.4A to D). Webs may be multiple and infrequently develop in the mid and lower esophagus.

Webs are common incidental findings, especially in middle-aged women. They may result from esophageal reflux or may be seen with increasing age. If the web is enough to cause dysphagia, being frequently fragile break down with the passage of an endoscope, or may require balloon dilatation. An association with the Plummer-Vinson syndrome has been described. The syndrome consists of iron-deficiency anemia, dysphagia, stomatitis, glossitis and koilonychia.

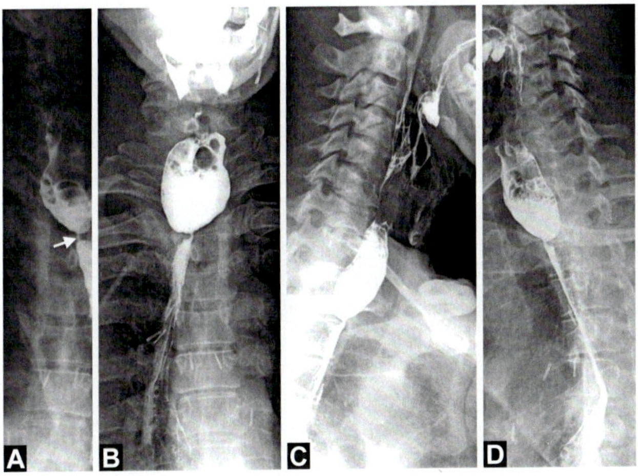

**Figs 5.4A to D:** A concentric upper esophageal webs seen in both the frontal and lateral projections (arrows). The way in which the web narrows the lumen is well seen in the lateral view

## DUODENAL ESOPHAGEAL ATRESIA

Esophageal and duodenal atresia have characteristic appearances on ultrasound, babies with duodenal atresia have slight distension of the upper abdomen as the stomach can decompress through the esophagus. When esophageal atresia coexists with duodenal atresia the stomach and duodenum are dilated due to the trapped gastric secretions. The abnormal degree of dilation allows discrimination from duodenal atresia.

New born baby presented with distended and palpable masses in upper abdomen with inability to pass a nasogastric tube. The kidigram shows gasless abdomen with coiling of nasogastric tube in upper thoracic region suggesting esophageal atresia. Ultrasound of abdomen shows fluid-filled stomach and duodenum. The ultrasound appearances suggest duodenal atresia associated with esophageal atresia. A confirmed case of duodenal esophageal atresia (Figs 5.5A to G) was subjected to duodeno-duodenostomy followed by esophageal repair at a later date.

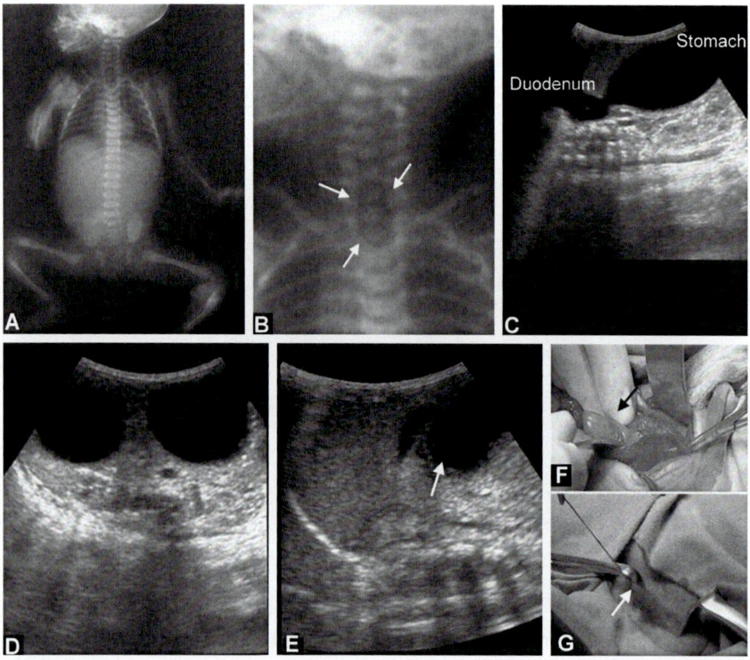


**Figs 5.5A to G:** Kidigram; (A) Magnified; (B) View reveals gasless abdomen and coiling of nasogastric tube in upper thoracic esophagus (arrows). Ultrasonography of abdomen in longitudinal; (C) Transverse; (D) Images reveals a dilated stomach and duodenum. Abrupt cut off of duodenum is well appreciated; (E) Intraoperative photographs reveal; (F) Distal end of duodenum (arrow); (G) Blind end of esophagus (arrow)

## ESOPHAGEAL DIVERTICULUM

Esophageal diverticulum is of little clinical significance. It develops in case with abnormal motility, most probably as a result of high intraluminal pressure. They are wide necked and are common at the level of the carina and lower esophagus (Figs 5.6A and B). Mid esophageal diverticula are produced by traction (traction diverticula) as a consequence of fibrosis from neighboring tuberculous lymph nodes.

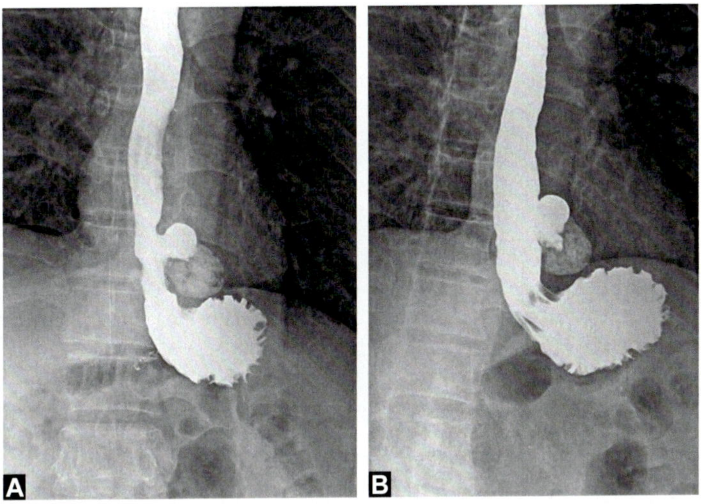


**Figs 5.6A and B:** 72 years old male on barium swallow shows wide neck esophageal diverticulum from lower third esophagus. The diverticulum at its dependant part contains food particles

## EPIGASTRIC HERNIA

Epigastric hernia is due to weakness in the abdominal muscle allowing the tissues of the abdomen to protrude through the muscle. Usually present at birth, and may heal without treatment as the infant grows and the abdominal muscles strengthen, it is a congenital hernia. Gastroschisis and omphalocele are other examples of congenital hernia.

### Causes

1. Increased intra-abdominal pressure
2. Weak abdominal wall
3. Obesity
4. Multiple pregnancies
5. Intra-abdominal masses

Typical locations of epigastric hernia are the points of weakness where no muscle is present, along the linea alba in the midline (Fig. 5.7).

When small only the peritoneum or the lining of the abdominal cavity may push through the muscle wall. In severe cases, portions of an organ may move through the hole in the muscle.

On ultrasound, seen in cross section, herniated bowel loops appear as target lesions with strong reflective central echoes representing air in the lumen, when obstructed they appear as tubular fluid filled structures containing valvulae conniventes or fecal material. Omentum may also herniate through the defect in anterior abdominal wall.

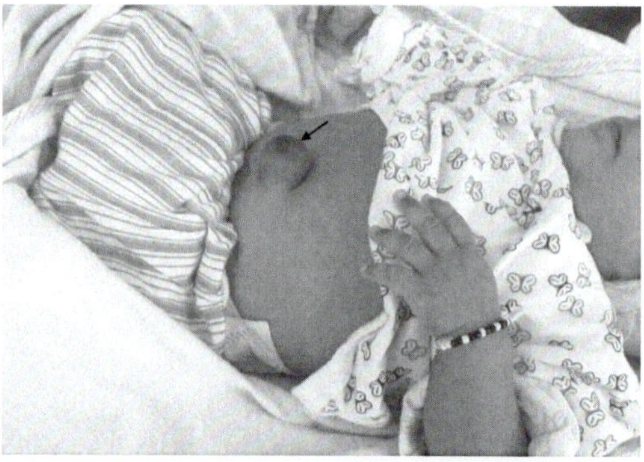

**Fig. 5.7:** Epigastric hernia seen in a three-months-old child (arrow)

## GASTROSCHISIS

Gastroschisis is congenital epigastric hernias (Fig. 5.8). It is a full thickness defect of the anterior abdominal wall, usually located to the right of umbilical cord. The defect is generally small and herniated organs include bowel loops and rarely liver. The other congenital epigastric hernias is omphalocele.

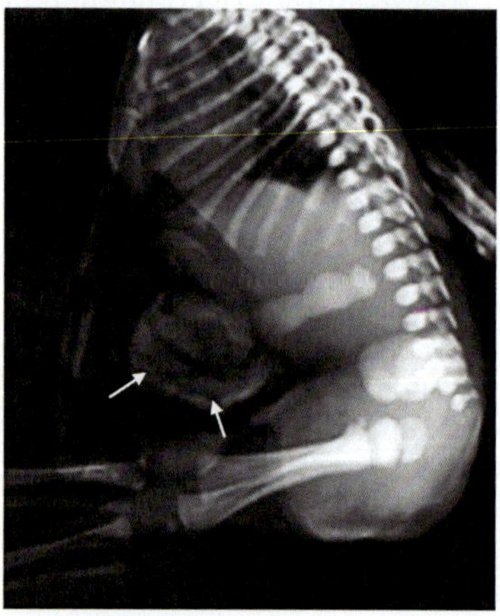

**Fig. 5.8:** Kidigram shows gastroschisis with herniation of bowel loops (arrow)

## EVENTRATION WITH MALROTATION OF MIDGUT

Elevation of a single hemidiaphragm is usually secondary to adjacent pleural, pulmonary, subphrenic disease or due to phrenic nerve palsy. Rarely, it is related to an intrinsic weakness of the diaphragm. In eventration weakened diaphragmatic muscles results in the upward displacement of abdominal contents but its incidence with malrotation of midgut is not seen. Occasionally, it is associated with superior renal ectopia as the kidney continues to migrate beyond the normal renal fossa (Figs 5.9A to C) during development and ends up in the thorax.

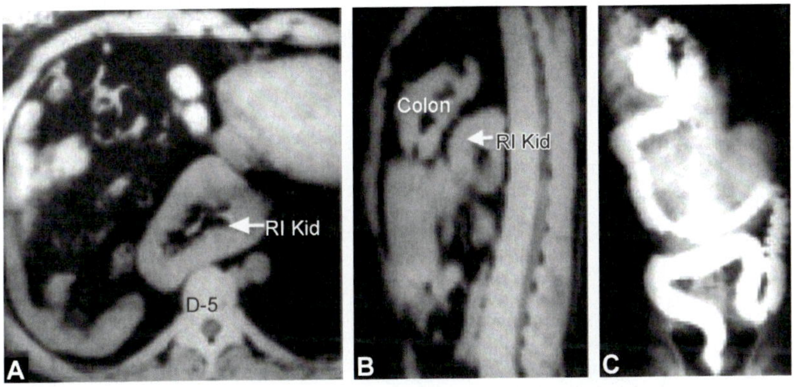


**Figs 5.9A to C:** (A) Axial CECT at chest level; (B) Sagittal reconstruction of chest and abdomen shows eventration of right hemidiaphragm with right kidney migrating into chest at D8 vertebral level; (C) Barium enema examination shows redundancy of the colon with ascending colon and cecum extending into the right hemithorax underlying the right hemidiaphragm. Upper GIT study (not in the figure) demonstrated the stomach in normal position with duodenojejunal flexure on the right side as part of malrotation of midgut (RI KID = right kidney)

## MECKEL'S DIVERTICULUM

Meckel's diverticulum measures 2 inches in length and is located within 2 feet of ileocecal valve on the antimesenteric border (Figs 5.10A and B). It occurs in 0.2 to 2% of population. It is a vestigial remnant of the omphalomesenteric duct. Majority are asymptomatic. If symptomatic generally presents before two years of age with painless rectal bleeding, intestinal obstruction, volvulus or intussusception. It may be present as an indirect hernia and is known as a "Hernia of Littre".

### Diagnosis

a. Approximately 50% of symptomatic Meckel's diverticula have ectopic gastric or pancreatic cells contained within it, the investigation of choice to diagnose Meckel's diverticula is nuclear scan with technetium-99m ($^{99m}$Tc) pertechnetate. It displays as a hot spot distant from the stomach as this scan detects gastric mucosa.
b. Small bowel follow through barium examination shows elongated, smoothly bordered, clublike, tubular structure arising from the distal ileum and lying parallel to its long axis.
c. On angiography presence of vitelline artery is pathognomonic.

Complications can be intestinal obstruction, peptic ulcer, perforation or diverticulitis.

Treatment is surgical resection.

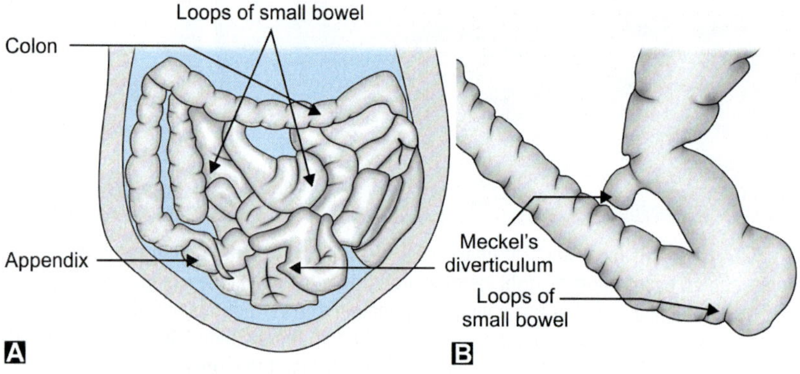


**Figs 5.10A and B:** Line diagram shows Meckel's diverticulum

## HIRSCHSPRUNG'S DISEASE

Hirschsprung's disease is due to arrest in the normal cranial-to-caudal neural cell migration, resulting in absence of ganglion cells within the myenteric plexus of the bowel wall. 70% of cases involve the rectosigmoid region. There is male predominance (4:1). A discrete zone of transition with a change in caliber of the bowel is more often seen in children than in the neonatal period (Figs 5.11A and B).

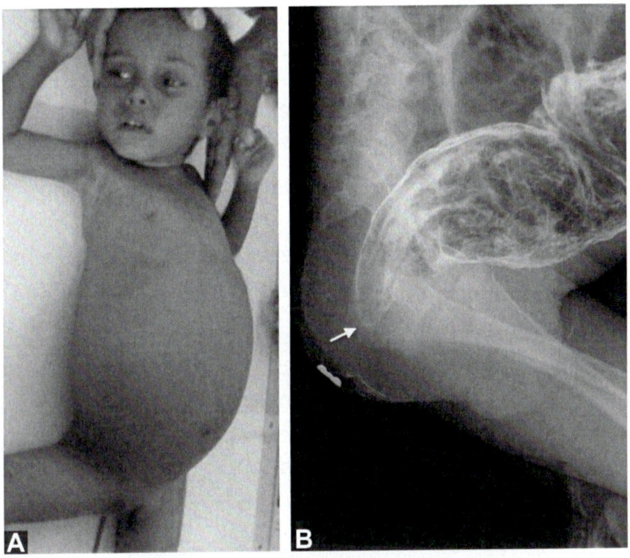

**Figs 5.11A and B:** Barium enema examination shows a discrete zone of transition (arrow) with abrupt increase in caliber of bowel in 5-year-old male presented with gross abdominal distension and failure to pass stool since a week

## IMPERFORATE ANUS/ANORECTAL MALFORMATION

Appearance of the perineum without an anal orifice is traditionally been referred to as imperforate anus. Now it is grouped under a generic term anorectal malformation (ARM). It is due to imperfect fusion of the post-allantoic gut with the proctodaeum. Incidence is one in 4500 births.

### Clinical Features

New born presents with inability to pass meconium, abdominal distension, intestinal obstruction, improper anal dimple and sometimes passing meconium per urethra.

It can be associated with VACTERL (vertebral, anorectal, cardiac, tracheoesophageal fistula, renal and limb anomalies) syndrome.

### Imaging Features

#### *Plain Radiography*

1. Prone cross table lateral view: This is the preferred projection because positioning is much easier and pitfalls of invertogram are avoided.

2. Wangentstein's invertogram: Usually done 6-12 hours after birth, so as to allow air to each the rectal pouch. A metal coin or marker is strapped at the presumed site of anus and X-ray is taken. Length between the rectal pouch and anal dimple marker is more than 2.5 cm in high imperforate anus. This can also be shown by an invertogram (Fig. 5.12)
   a. In low fistula, rectal pouch is distal to the Stephern's line (Pubococcygeal line).
   b. In intermediate, pouch is at the level of ischial spine (Kelly's point).
   c. In high fistula, rectal pouch is proximal to the Stephen's line.
3. USG abdomen plays role in detecting associated anomalies of the genitourinary system and congenital heart diseases and to assess the distance of rectal pouch in relation to the surface of perineum.
4. MRI spine in selected cases is necessary to make a definite diagnosis of tethered cord or other spinal abnormalities. It is also used to define the anatomy of pelvic muscles.

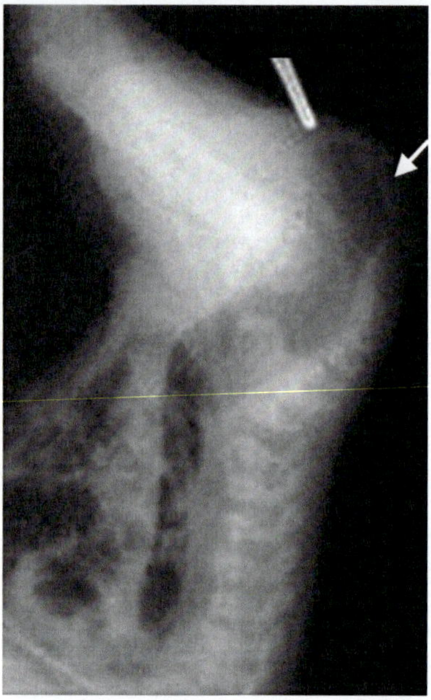

Fig. 5.12: X-ray invertogram shows the marker is at the site of anus and X-ray is taken. Length between the air column rectum and anal dimple marker is less than 2.5 cm, it is low imperforate anus

### Treatment

1. In low imperforate anus, single stage reconstruction is done under general anesthesia with very good results.
   i. Anoplasty
   ii. Anovestibuloplasty
   iii. Anal dilatation
   iv. Incision of anal membrane
2. In high imperforate anus, initial colostomy is done. Later definitive procedure, i.e. pull through operation through puborectalis and anastomosis of rectal pouch to create the anal canal is done. Closure of colostomy is done later.

   Posterior sagittal anorectoplasty is commonly done procedure.

### Complications

- Infection
- Fecal fistula
- Stenosis
- Colitis
- Malnutrition
- Fecal incontinence

## TERTIARY CONTRACTIONS (ABNORMAL MOTILITY) IN ESOPHAGUS

Tertiary contractions are seen as intermittent ripples along the wall of the esophagus and are seen as multiple instantaneous contraction rings. The barium column appears segmented producing a corkscrew appearance (Figs 5.13A to D). Tertiary contractions may last only few seconds.

In young adults most swallows will be entirely normal but with age the proportion of abnormal swallows increase. Primary and secondary waves become weak, sometimes failing to clear the esophagus of the bolus, the peristaltic wave may fail to run the complete length of the esophagus and the lower esophageal sphincter may on occasions fail to relax and result in tertiary contractions which become more frequent.

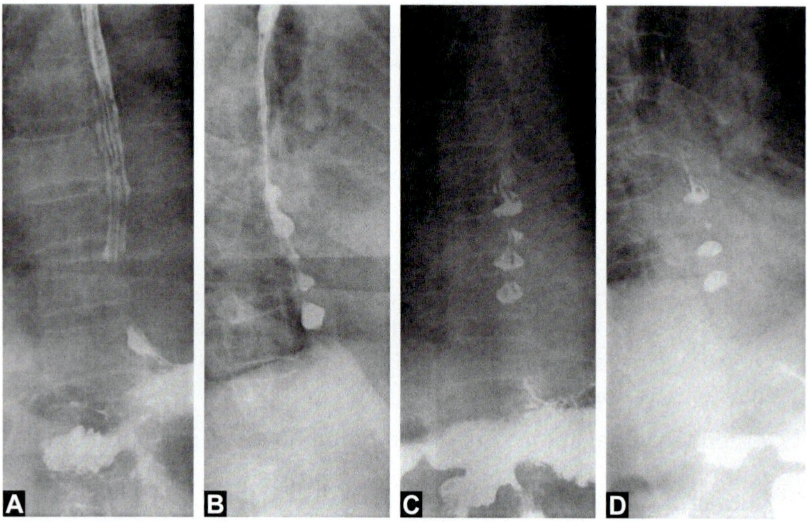

Figs 5.13A to D: Barium swallow in a 66 years old male shows tertiary contractions of the esophagus seen as a series of indentations resembling a corkscrew, there by called corkscrew esophagus

## ROUNDWORM INFESTATION

A variety of parasites may dwell in the small bowel. Ascaris lumbricoides is a roundworm infestation which is extremely widespread. Infestation involves the small bowel, liver and lungs. The worm can migrate to the biliary tree, pharynx and nasal cavity. In small bowel they may be so abundant and may result in intestinal obstruction. On barium examination once the roundworms has swallowed contrast; the barium is seen within their intestinal tract (Fig. 5.14).

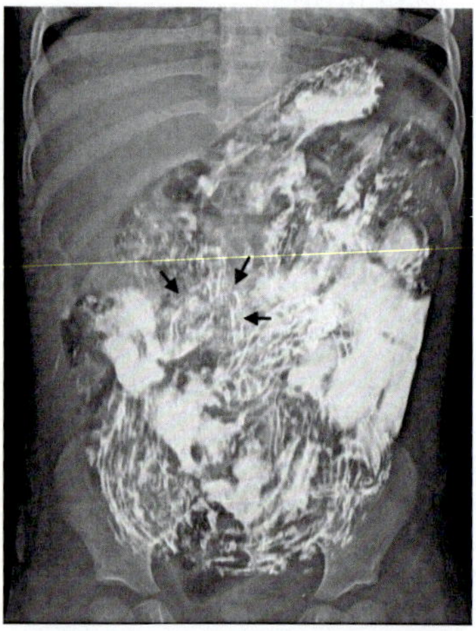

Fig. 5.14: Barium meal examination shows multiple round worms in the small intestine

Other parasites that may dwell in the gut are hookworm, tapeworm and strongyloides which present with vague findings of mucosal thickening, nodularity, mild dilatation and flocculation on contrast examination.

## TRICHOBEZOAR

Bezoar is a collection of undigested material that is unable to leave the stomach. Most bezoars comprise of indigestible organic matter, when this matter consists of hair it is called trichobezoars and if it consist of fibers of vegetable and fruit it is called phytobezoars.

Trichobezoars, commonly occur in patients with psychiatric disturbances who chew and swallow their own hair. They may have vague symptoms ranging from abdominal mass to gastrointestinal symptoms.

Barium meal examination shows a mobile, intraluminal filling defects with barium filled mottled appearance (Fig. 5.15). CT gives mottled appearance with oral contrast or may sometimes give a concentric ring appearance free from stomach wall.

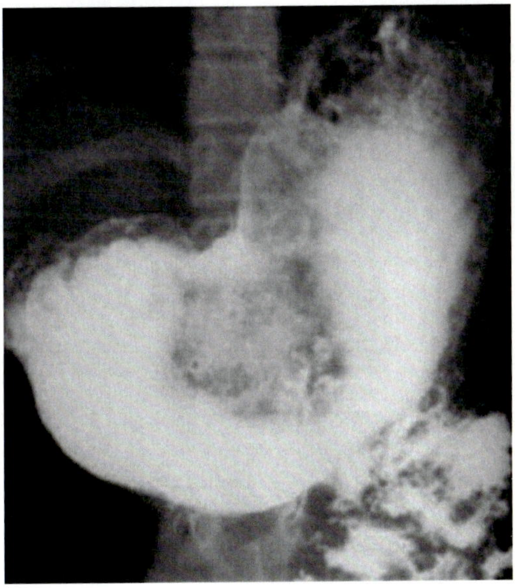

Fig. 5.15: Barium meal examination shows a large intraluminal filling defects with barium filled mottled appearance

Complications can be mechanical obstruction of small bowel and rarely perforation and peritonitis. A trichobezoar which extends into the small bowel is called as Rapunzel syndrome. Treatment for a small trichobezoar is endoscopic removal by laparoscopy and if large by surgery.

In children bezoar can occur rarely in the colon or rectum (Figs 5.16A to C). It is generally followed by consumption of watermelon seeds, pumpkin seeds, prickly pear seeds or salted sunflower seeds with shells. Children with rectal bezoars typically present with diarrhea, rectal or abdominal pain, tenesmus, fever and vomiting.

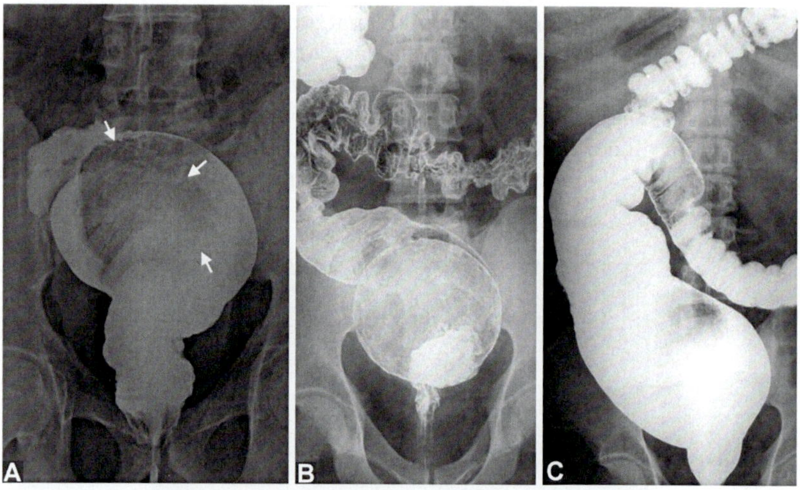

**Figs 5.16A to C:** Barium enema examination shows a rounded intraluminal filling defects (arrows) in the rectum, a rectal bezoar

## INTUSSUSCEPTION

Intussusception is the telescoping of one segment of bowel into the adjacent segment. The prolapsed segment is called intussusceptum while the receiving segment is the intussuscipient. Ileocolic intussusception is common in children; it commonly affects children less than 2 years of age and is more common in boys. Ileoileocolic, colocolic and ileoileal intussesceptions are less common.

Most intussusceptions are idiopathic thought to be due to inflammation and edema of Peyer's patches. Other causes are Meckel's diverticulum, duplication cysts, lymphoma, polyps, and hematoma.

Apex and inner tubes will have compromised blood supply which leads to gangrene. Apex sloughs off and bleeds which mixes with the mucus to produce the classic red currant jelly passed per anus. Perforation and peritonitis may be secondary to gangrene.

The classical triad of abdominal pain, currant jelly stools and palpable abdominal mass is seen in less than 50 per cent of cases. On examination, a sausage shaped mass is felt on either side of umbilicus with concavity towards umbilicus. Often mass appears and disappears.

USG is the initial investigation of choice. It shows a mass with either an atypical target or a concentric ring appearance in transverse section and sandwich/pseudo-kidney appearance in sagittal plane. Eccentric, semilunar, echogenic mesenteric fat is seen on transverse section that is pulled along with the vessels and lymph nodes into the intussusceptions.

On color Doppler imaging absence of blood flow might indicate the presence of ischemia or necrosis.

Plain film findings are nonspecific. Soft-tissue mass in the region of cecum or transvers colon with meniscus sign may be seen with absence of cecal gas or stool. Features of small bowel obstruction may be seen.

On barium enema study an intussusception is seen as a convex intraluminal filling defect. Coiled spring appearance may be produced as the contrast insinuates between the intussusceptum and the intussuscipiens. CT abdomen (Fig. 5.17) shows evidence of bowel within bowel appearance of small bowel in paraumbilical region giving 'Target' appearance with surrounding dilated fecal filled large bowel loops.

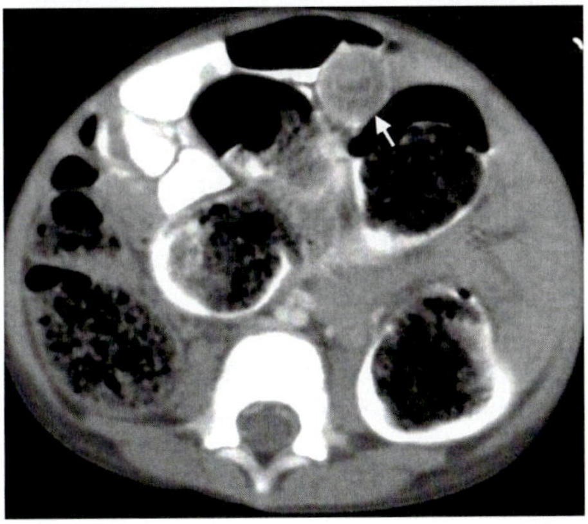

Fig. 5.17: CT abdomen in a 3 years old child shows evidence of bowel within bowel appearance of small bowel in paraumbilical region giving 'Target' appearance - suggestive of ileoileal intussusception. Dilated fecal filled large bowel loops are seen

Initial treatment starts with Ryle's tube aspiration, IV fluids and antibiotic. After stabilization of the child, reduction can be attempted using either dilute barium or water soluble contrast or more recently using air under either fluoroscopic or US guidance. Successful reduction is marked by free flow of contrast into the terminal ileum with disappearance of soft tissue mass.

Surgery is indicated if initial treatment fails and more than 48 hours have passed and on development of features of perforation, peritonitis or strangulation.

## APPENDICITIS

### Introduction

The appendix is a blind-ending tubular structure arising from the cecum. Appendicitis is acute inflammation of the appendix and the most common abdominal surgical emergency (Figs 5.18A and B).

It occurs in all age groups but is rare in infants; the incidence becomes increasingly common in childhood, reaching a peak incidence in the late teenage years and early 20's. The mean age when appendicitis occurs in the pediatric population is 6-10 years.

It may be complicated by perforation. An inflamed or perforated appendix can be walled off by the adjacent greater omentum or small-bowel loops, resulting in phlegmonous appendicitis or focal abscess. Abscess may be intraperitoneal or retroperitoneal. It is most often located in the proximity of the appendix, so that the inflammatory mass usually lies adjacent to cecum and terminal ileum in right iliac fossa. When the appendix is abnormally located or is unusually long the abscesses have been described in the left lower quadrant, the right flank, anterior abdominal wall, the lesser sac, and subhepatic and subdiaphragmatic spaces.

### Imaging

On plain abdominal radiograph the findings are nonspecific and often non contributary. When abscess is present, it shows a poorly defined mass, with displacement of a adjacent loops of bowel. Irregular radiolucencies in the mass are due to bubbles of gas giving a mottled pattern. In some cases the abscess may form a unilocular mass containing gas or pus with fluid level.

On barium studies non filling of appendix is associated with an external or intramural mass indenting medial aspect of cecum. Terminal ileum may be displaced or narrowed by the adjacent inflammatory mass, thickening of the mucosal folds.

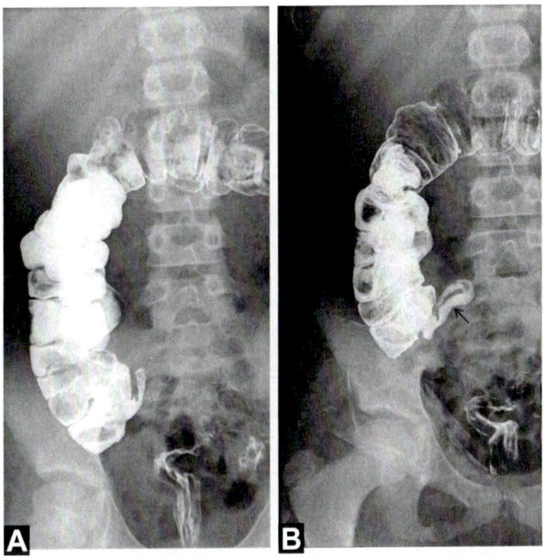


**Figs 5.18A and B:** Normal appendix in two different patients on barium enema examination

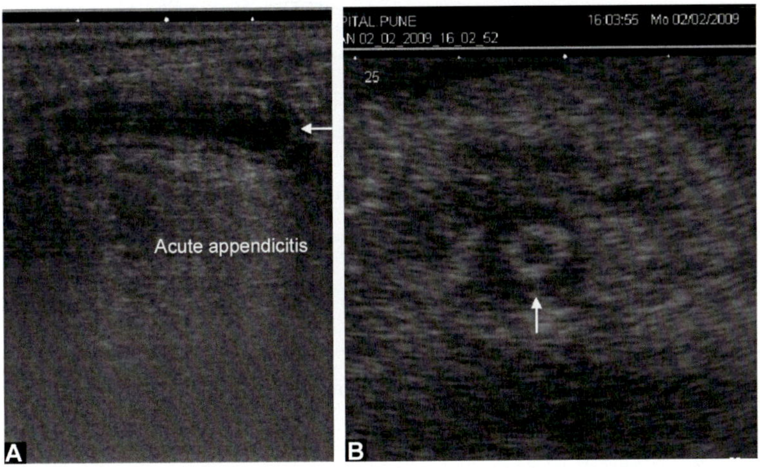


**Figs 5.19A and B:** USG right iliac fossa (A) Long section; (B) Cross section of inflamed appendix

On USG Puylaert's technique of using graded compression is a popular method. It shows mixed echogenic mass in the region of the appendix with thickened paracecal mass (Figs 5.19A and B). Liquefaction and abscess formation will manifest as fluid component. Gas bubbles may be seen within the mass. Doppler study shows presence of hyperemia in the appendiceal wall and adjacent meso-appendix.

CT is particularly useful where appendiceal perforation is suspected. The diagnostic accuracy remains high and is also useful for characterizing periappendiceal inflammatory masses.

Associated findings are extraluminal air, marked ileocecal thickening, localized lymphadenopathy and small bowel obstruction.

## RICHTER'S HERNIA

Richter's hernia occurs when the antimesenteric wall of the intestine protrudes through a defect in the abdominal wall (Fig. 5.20). It is a relatively uncommon but hazardous type of hernia.

If such a herniation becomes necrotic and is subsequently reduced during hernia repair, perforation and peritonitis may result.

A Richter's hernia can result in strangulation and necrosis in the absence of intestinal obstruction.

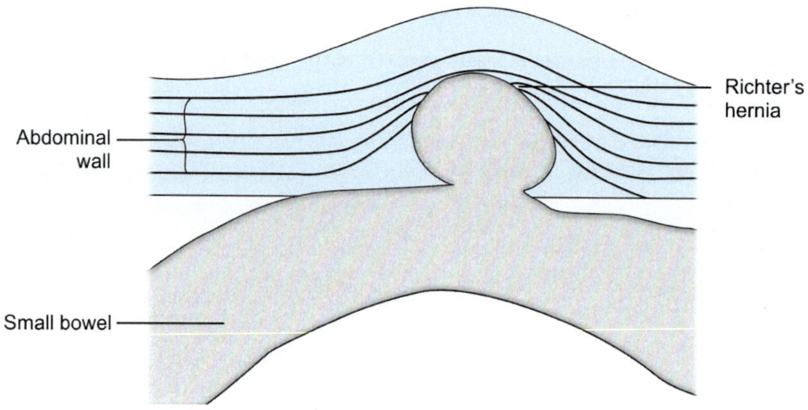


**Fig. 5.20:** Line diagram shows Richter's hernia

## COLONIC DIVERTICULOSIS

A diverticulum is a saclike protrusion in the colonic wall that develops as a result of herniation of the mucosa and submucosa through point of weakness in the muscular wall of the colon. The colonic diverticulum is a false or pulsion diverticulum, that is, it does not contain all layers of the colonic wall. Diverticulosis indicates the presence of multiple diverticula which are demonstrated on a barium enema study (Fig. 5.21). Diverticulitis describes the presence of an inflammatory process associated with diverticula. Its pathogenesis is attributed to genetic and environmental factors.

A barium enema examination should be avoided in acute presentations in patients with suspected acute diverticulitis and localized peritoneal signs because of a possible extravasation of barium into the peritoneal cavity, which can increase the morbidity and mortality related to barium-induced chemical peritonitis. Abdominal ultrasound is helpful, especially in female patients, to exclude pelvic and gynecological pathology. CT is generally superior to barium studies.

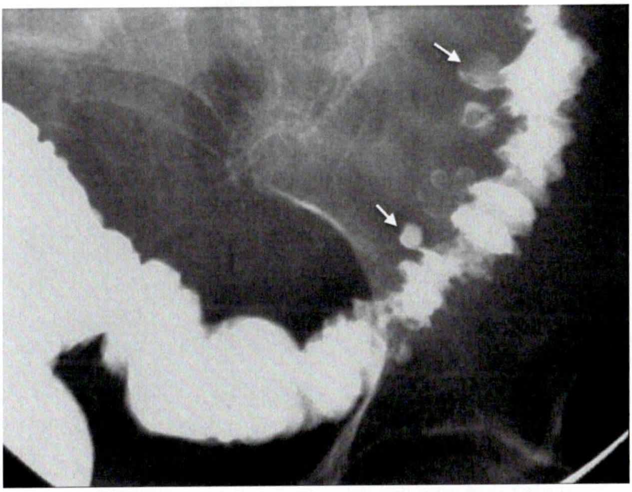

**Fig. 5.21:** Barium enema examination shows diverticulosis in descending colon (arrow)

## ILLEOCECAL TUBERCULOSIS

The illeocecal region is the most common site of intestinal tuberculosis because of abundant lymphoid tissue, physiological stasis and increased rate of absorption. The lesion can be ulcerative, hyperplastic, or ulcerohyperplastic with short annular defect and overhanging edges.

In ileocecal tuberculosis the barium meal follow through or entroclysis followed by barium enema is the imaging modality of choice. In equivocal cases CT is resorted to.

## Barium Study

Thickening of ileocecal valve lips with narrowing of the terminal ileum is characteristic of tuberculosis (Figs 5.22A and B) called as Fleischer sign. The double contrast barium enema study shows shallow ulcer with elevated margins, linear or stellate in configuration and follow orientation of lymphoid follicles (longitudinal in ileum and transverse in colon). Fold thickening, contour irregularity and skip lesions may be seen.

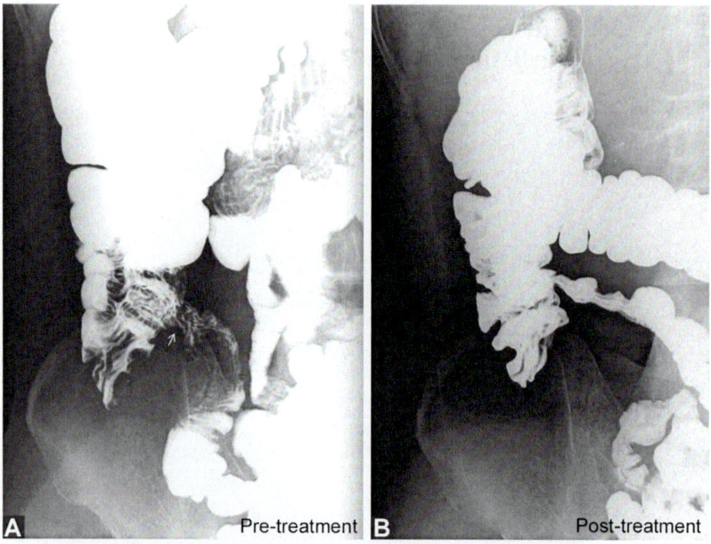


**Figs 5.22A and B:** Barium meal follow through examination in a case of ileocecal tuberculosis: (A) Pre-treatment study that the cecum is shrunken, conical and lifted superiorly due to contraction of mesocolon; (B) After treatment there is improvement in filling of terminal ileum and cecum

The cecum classically becomes shrunken, conical, tapering and withdrawn out of the iliac fossa due to contraction of mesocolon. Hepatic flexure may be pulled down. There is loss of normal illeo cecal angle and the dilated terminal ileum may appear hanging from the pulled up, shortened cecum (Figs 5.23A to C). The illeocecal valve becomes fixed, irregular, incompetent rigid and obliterated cecum is called as Stierlin's sign.

CT may show circumferential wall thickening in terminal ileum and cecum measuring up to 3 cm in diameter. There is asymmetrical thickening of ileocecal valve and medial wall of cecum with the wall thickening extending into the terminal ileum. There may be adjacent mesenteric lymphadenopathy. The differential diagnosis is with Crohn's disease in which there is uniform concentric wall thickening with symmetrical mural stratification which is not seen in tuberculosis.

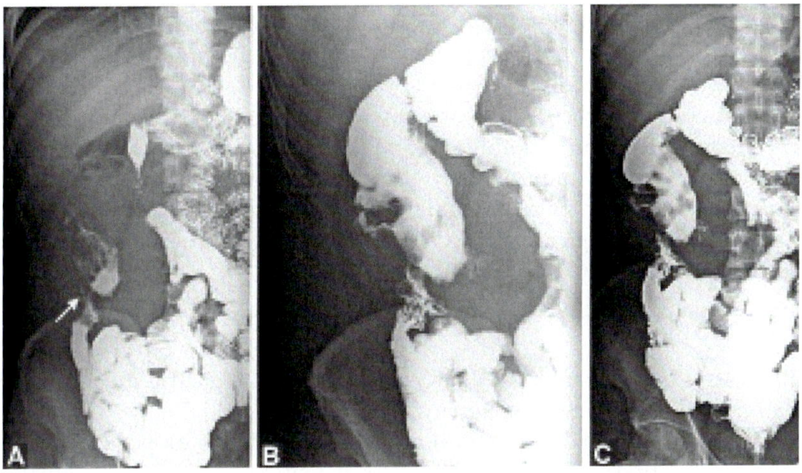


**Figs 5.23A to C:** Barium meal follow through examination shows thickening of ileocecal valve lips with narrowing of the terminal ileum in a case of ileocecal tuberculosis

## ANAL FISSURE

An anal fissure is synonymous with fissure-in-ano. It is an elongated ulcer in the long axis of the lower anal canal. It is one of the most painful conditions resulting in a lot of discomfort and embarrassment to the patient. Bleeding occurs at the end of defecation.

Predisposing factors are: Constipation, irregularity of diet, consumption of spicy and pungent food, faulty bowel habits, and lack of local hygiene and pregnancy.

### Chronic or Complicated Fissure-in-ano

The fissure is labeled as chronic or complicated if it fulfils the following criteria. If not responding to conservative treatment.

1. If a fibrous anal polyp is present.
2. Presence of an external skin tag is noticed.
3. Presence of hemorrhoid is visible.
4. If there is exposure of the fibers of the internal sphincter at the floor of the fissure.

5. The base of fissure is infected.
6. A bridged fissure with underlying fistula (a post fissure fistula) is diagnosed.

Treatment of superficial fissures is by: Warm water Sitz bath, adequate analgesia, stool softening, high-fiber-diet and bulk-forming agents and reassurance and encouragement for not resisting the urge for defecation help prevent hard stools.

Treatments of chronic fissures available are: Local application of vasodilators, injection of botulinum toxin, oral nifedipine, endoscopic anal dilatation, chemical cauterization, excision of the anal fissure (fissurectomy), fissurectomy with immediate skin grafting, division of internal anal sphincter, surgical and cyrotherapeutical treatment and carbon dioxide laser surgery.

## GASTRIC ULCER

The gastric ulcer is an inflammatory erosion of the gastric mucosa. The ulcer may be benign and malignant.

The benign ulcer is located along lesser curvature or posterior wall of antrum or body. The malignant ulcer is usually located along greater curvature.

The imaging modalities include barium meal examination, CT and virtual gastroscopy.

The findings in barium meal study are as per Table 5.1 (Figs 5.24A and B).

**Table 5.1:** Findings in gastric ulcer on barium meal study

| Benign ulcer | Malignant ulcer |
|---|---|
| The ulcer project beyond the gastric wall. | The ulcer does not project beyond the expected gastric contour. |
| Ulcer crater is seen as round or ovoid collection of barium. | The ulcer crater with radiolucent elevated border is called as 'Carman meniscus'sign. |
| The Hamptons line is the radiolucent line separating barium in gastric lumen and barium in crater.<br>The ulcer mound is seen as smooth bilobed hemispherical mass projecting in the lumen on both sides of the ulcer. The outer border forms obtuse, gently sloping angles with adjacent gastric wall. | Discrete tumor mass seen forming acute angle with gastric wall. |
| The ulcer coller is the radiolucent rim of edema around the ulcer. | Nodular, clubbed, fused or amputed folds are seen. |

The contrast enhanced CT with oral water soluble contrast may show ulcer as an out pouching. The associated signs include wall thickening and luminal narrowing of the stomach, sub mucous edema, infiltration of surrounding fat, pancreas, liver. Enlarged lymph nodes and liver metastasis can be seen in malignant ulcer.

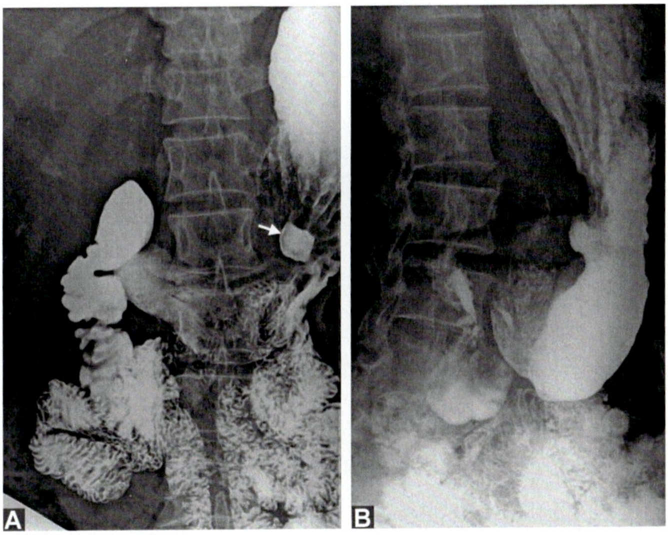


**Figs 5.24A and B:** Gastric ulcer is located in the posterior wall with ulcer crater seen enface (A) with mucosal folds extending up to the edge off ulcer crater. In profile (B) The ulcer is seen to protrude outside the expected line of stomach wall

## DUODENAL ULCER

Duodenal ulcer is mucosal erosion of duodenum. Ninety five percent are bulbar ulcers (Fig. 5.25) while 5% are post bulbar. Bulbar ulcer can be seen at apex, central portion or base of the bulb while post bulbar is seen on medial wall of proximal descending duodenum. Ulcer more than 2 cm in diameter is referred as giant duodenal ulcer and if present is always located in the duodenal bulb.

The imaging modality of choice is double contrast barium meal examination. The findings include persistent, small, ovoid or linear barium collection or ulcer niche with smooth edematous mucosal, folds converging centrally at the edge of ulcer crater. The barium coating rim of unfilled ulcer crater is seen as ring shadow in double contrast view. The other findings include deformity of the duodenal bulb.

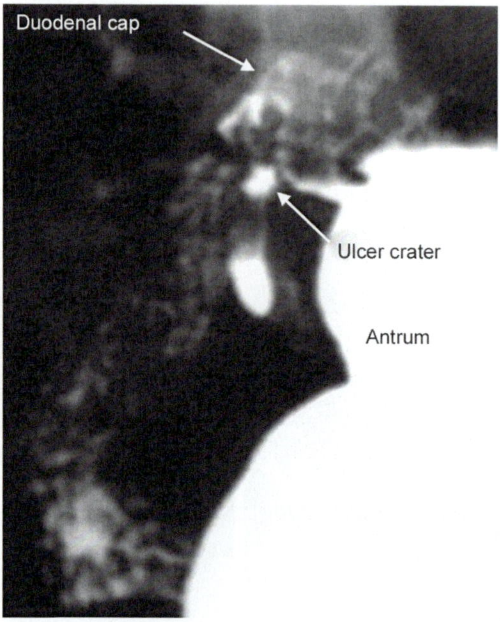


Fig. 5.25: Barium meal examination shows duodenal ulcer

## CARCINOMA ESOPHAGUS

Sixty percent of esophageal carcinomas are of squamous cell type (Figs 5.26A and B). They are equally distributed throughout the length of the esophagus and forty per cent are adenocarcinomas which occur in the lower esophagus (Figs 5.26C and D) from dysplasia of metaplastic columnar epithelium that has developed as a result of longstanding reflux esophagitis.

The majority of patients with esophageal carcinoma presenting with dysphagia already have tumor that has spread to involve regional lymph-nodes, so the prognosis is poor. The tumor mass with or without enlarged local lymph nodes may produce a mediastinal mass on X-ray chest.

Barium swallow frequently shows irregular narrowing of lumen with shouldering (Figs 5.26A to D) effect and rolled margins. Endoscopy and biopsy should always be performed.

Contrast-enhanced CT (CECT) chest shows circumferential wall thickening of esophagus with loss of fat planes with bronchus, pulmonary artery and aorta with narrowing of the esophageal lumen (Figs 5.27A and B).

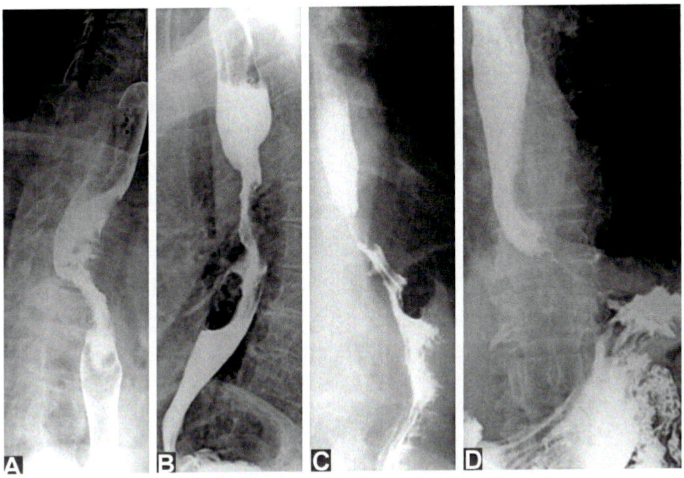


**Figs 5.26A to D:** Barium meal examination of four different cases of esophageal carcinoma show middle third involvement in A and B and involvement of lower esophagus in C and D. The lesions show irregular narrowing of lumen with shouldering effect and rolled margins

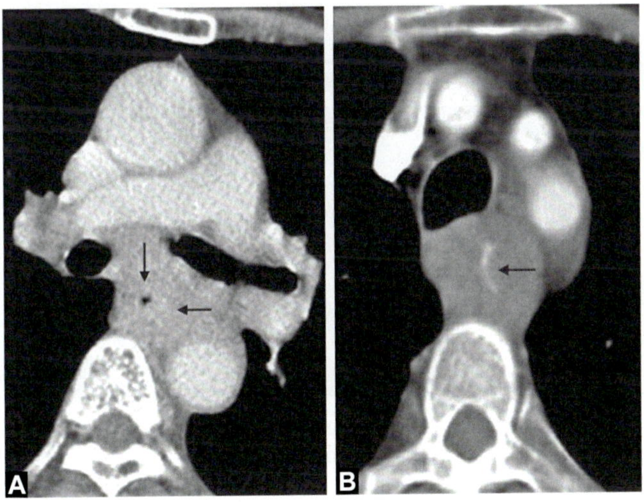


**Figs 5.27A and B:** Contrast-enhanced CT (CECT) chest shows (A) Circumferential wall thickening of mid esophagus with loss of fat planes with bronchus, pulmonary artery and aorta. The esophageal lumen is narrowed. Contrast-enhanced CT in another case shows; (B) Well-defined asymmetric circumferential wall thickening of the esophagus in midthoracic region causing marked luminal narrowing

## MALIGNANCY STOMACH

Atrophic gastritis predisposes to the development of carcinoma stomach. A sequence of events which may follow atrophic gastritis are development of intestinal metaplasia, dysplasia and to neoplasia. Malignancy involving the distal antrum often gives an apple core contour (Figs 5.28A to D) which can be mistaken for the normal pyloric canal if the tumor joins with the pyloric canal.

When permeation of the growth becomes extensive, the stomach develops appearance of a leather bottle or "linitis plastica". Carcinoma of the fundus may infiltrate submucosally into the distal esophagus to produce a look that imitates achalasia cardia.

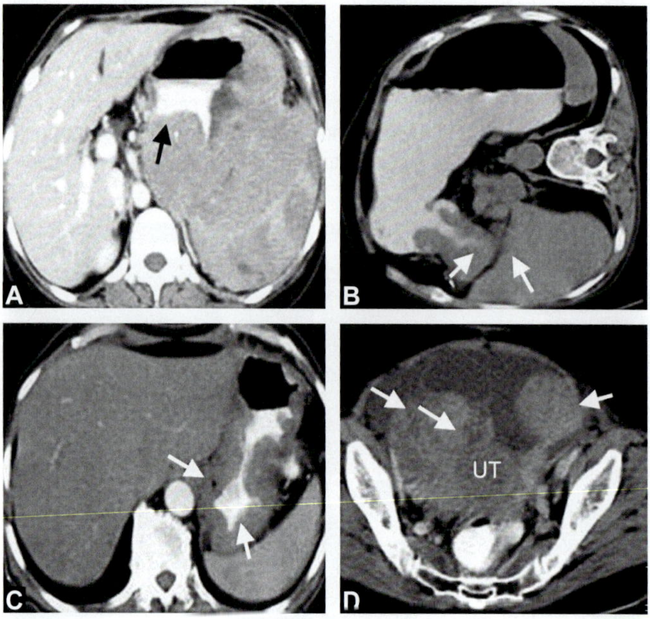


**Figs 5.28A to D:** (A) CT shows diffuse thickening of walls of stomach with narrowing of lumen in a case of gastric lymphoma; (B) CT image in right lateral recumbent position shows circumferential thickening of pylorus with the growth extending into antrum and duodenum. Prepyloric lymph node is seen (arrow) in a case of carcinoma of the pylorus; (C) Homogeneously enhancing circumferential thickening of almost the entire stomach wall is seen in this case of carcinoma of stomach. Few enlarged lymph nodes are also present; (D) Ascites and bilateral ovarian deposits (Krukenberg tumor) in a previously operated case of carcinoma stomach

## BOWEL ISCHEMIA

Bowel ischemia is hypoxia of the small bowel or colon. Bowel ischemia is characterized by inadequate blood flow to or from the involved mesenteric vessels supplying a particular segment of bowel. The organs typically affected are the small bowel or colon as a result of inadequate. Blood supply, the cause can be occlusive or non-occlusive. The ischemia can be acute or chronic.

Plain radiographic abdomen findings are often normal, may show similar irregularity as seen on barium study (Fig. 5.29A). Barium enema examination, shows irregular bowel lumen giving a thumb printing appearance (Fig. 5.29B).

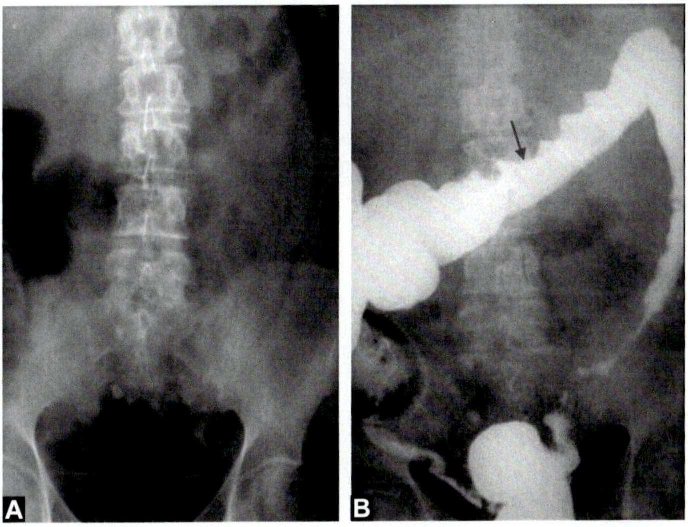


**Figs 5.29A and B:** Plain film and barium study showing thumb printing (arrow) suggestive of bowel ischemia

CT is the primary imaging modality and it has been proven to be highly accurate. CT scans shows mesenteric edema with irregular thickening of the wall of the small or large bowel that is greater than 3 mm and 5 mm respectively. With proper timing of the contrast-agent bolus, a thrombus in a large vessel can be seen as a soft-tissue filling defect (Figs 5.30A and B). Angiography reveals the site of arterial occlusion of a diseased bowel segment.

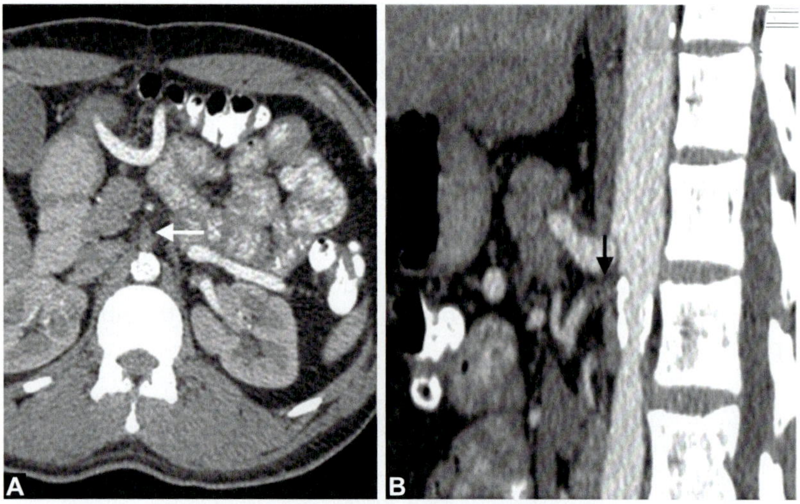

**Figs 5.30A and B:** Contrast enhanced CT shows thrombosis of the SMA (arrow) in both A and B

# 6 CHAPTER

# Hepatobiliary System, Pancreas and Spleen

Chapter Outline



## SIMPLE HEPATIC CYST

Liver cysts are benign congenital malformations resulting from isolated aberrant biliary ducts. The cyst contents are usually clear serous fluid. They do not invade biliary or vascular elements, but may cause obstruction or compression atrophy of the liver parenchyma when they attain a large size (Figs 6.1A and B). Complications are hemorrhage, rupture, torsion and infection.

## AMEBIC LIVER ABSCESS

Amebic liver abscess is the most common extra intestinal manifestation of amebiasis. It is caused by the protozoan *Entamoeba histolytica*. The protozoan reaches the liver by penetrating through the colon, invading the mesenteric venules and entering the portal vein. It may reach by means of lymphatics or directly enter the liver from the hepatic flexure. As the liver

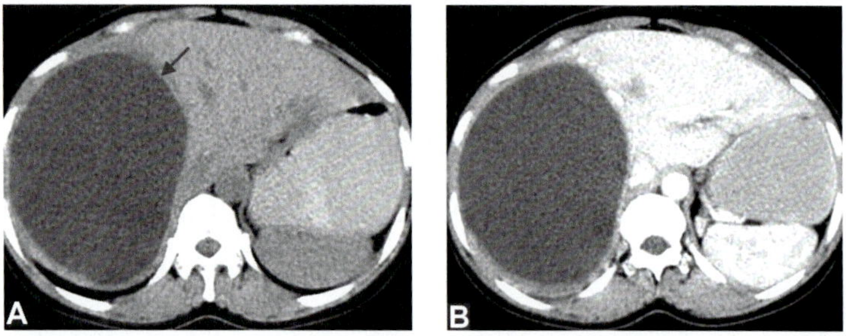


**Figs 6.1A and B:** (A) Plain; (B) Contrast CT abdomen show a large thin walled hypodense (12 HU) cystic lesion in the liver with smooth margins. No septae or calcifications seen

tissue is destroyed it develops into an abscess filled with thick fluid which resembles anchovy sauce. Abscess is generally located in the right lobe of liver. The abscess may be single or multiple.

Chest X-ray may show elevation of the right dome of diaphragm, small right pleural effusion or right lower lobe atelectasis. Abdominal radiographs may show hepatomegaly. Intrahepatic gas or an air fluid level can occur in case percutaneous aspiration has been carried out or secondary infection by gas producing organisms has taken place.

Ultrasound examination shows a round or oval lesion having poor echogenicity as compared to normal liver and absence of a prominent abscess wall with posterior acoustic enhancement, it may contain few low level internal echoes.

On CT amebic abscesses of the liver appear as low attenuation lesions, the density of the lesion depends on its stage of development and internal contents. It is surrounded by peripheral rim which is isodense to hypodense on unenhanced CT scans and usually enhances after contrast administration (Figs 6.2A and B). Amebic abscess should be included in the differential diagnosis when CT shows one or more cystic or complex lesion within the liver, especially when there is evidence of extrahepatic extension. The presence of pleural effusion and or perihepatic fluid in association with a cystic or complex hepatic mass is certainly not specific for amebic abscess and can be seen with many inflammatory and neoplastic hepatic lesions.

## Complications Include

1. Pleuropulmonary amebiasis is the most frequent complication of amebic liver abscess, and manifest as pulmonary consolidation, abscess, serous effusion, empyema or hepatobronchial fistula.
2. Intraperitoneal rupture of hepatic abscess.

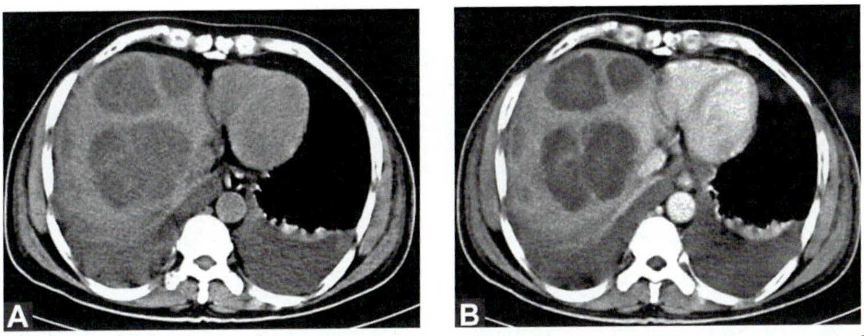


**Figs 6.2A and B:** (A) Plain; (B) Contrast CT abdomen shows multiple, irregular, hypodense lesions with minimally enhancing thin walls and mild perilesional edema in the enlarged liver. Reactionary bilateral pleural effusion and ascites are seen. Aspirate had anchovy sauce appearance

3. Rupture into the pericardium is the most serious complication.
4. Abscess may develop a biliary communication.

Management by medical therapy may be instituted using either a single agent or a combination of drugs for the extraluminal parasite. Amebicidal drugs may be classified into 3 groups : luminal, tissue, and mixed amebicides.

Aspiration or drainage of abscess should be done in all situations on failure of medical treatment to show clinical improvement in 48 to 72 hours.

Open surgical drainage may be required in the setting of a large abscess with a poor yield on needle aspiration or clinical deterioration despite attempted needle aspiration and in complicated amebic liver abscesses.

## HEPATIC CIRRHOSIS

Cirrhosis results from chronic liver disease characterized by replacement of liver tissue by fibrosis, scar tissue and regenerative nodules leading to loss of liver function. Alcoholism, hepatitis and fatty liver are the common etiological factors (Figs 6.3A and B).

Imaging includes ultrasound, CT and MR. The finding in advanced cirrhosis is atrophy of the posterior segments of the right lobe (VI and VII), hypertrophy of the caudate lobe (I) and of lateral segments of the left lobe (II and III). The cause of this is increased hepatic blood flow in certain areas and decreased hepatic blood flow in some.

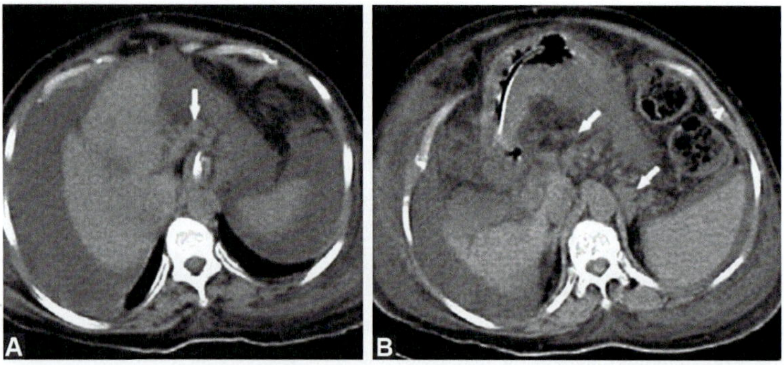


**Figs 6.3Aand B:** Shrunken liver with nodular contour, esophageal and splenoportal collaterals (arrow) are seen along with massive ascites indicating portal hypertension

The ultrasound findings include nodular, coarse liver parenchyma with increased echogenicity, atrophy of right lobe, hypertrophy of the caudate lobe and of lateral segments of the left lobe. The color Doppler reveals hepatofugal flow in portal hypertension.

The CT scan also shows splenomegaly and vascular derangements in the form of varices, arterioportal and porto-venous shunts. The cirrhosis induced hepatocellular carcinoma shows heterogeneous mass having arterial enhancement with early washout.

The MR shows signal intensities on T1 and T2-weighted images as follows:

| LESION | T1W | T2W |
|---|---|---|
| Regenerative nodule | hypointense | hypointense |
| Dysplastic nodule | hyperintense | hypointense |
| HCC nodule | hypointense | hyperintense |
| Fatty change | hyperintense | hypointense |
| Fibrotic change | hypointense | hyperintense |

## HEPATIC TRAUMA

Liver is the second most frequently injured abdominal organ (Table 6.1). Posterior segment of right lobe is most frequent site (near spine and ribs). Lacerations extending to bare area may only have retroperitoneal finding (Figs 6.4A to D).

**Table 6.1:** Grades of liver injury

| | |
|---|---|
| Grade 1 | Subcapsular hematoma, less than 10% of surface area. Laceration capsular tear, less than 1 cm parenchymal depth. |
| Grade 2 | Hematoma subcapsular, 10-50% surface area. Intraparenchymal hematoma, less than 10 cm in diameter. Laceration 1-3 cm parenchymal depth, less than 10 cm in length. |
| Grade 3 | Subcapsular hematoma, more than 50% of surface area or expanding. Ruptured subcapsular or parenchymal hematoma. Intraparenchymal hematoma more than 10 cm or expanding. Laceration more than 3 cm in parenchymal depth. |
| Grade 4 | Laceration with parenchymal disruption involving 25-75% of a hepatic lobe or one to three of Couinaud's segments in a single lobe. |
| Grade 5 | Laceration with parenchymal disruption involving more than 75% of hepatic lobe or more than three of Couinaud's segments in a single lobe. |
| Grade 6 | Vascular juxtahepatic venous injuries (i.e. retrohepatic vena cava or central major hepatic veins). |

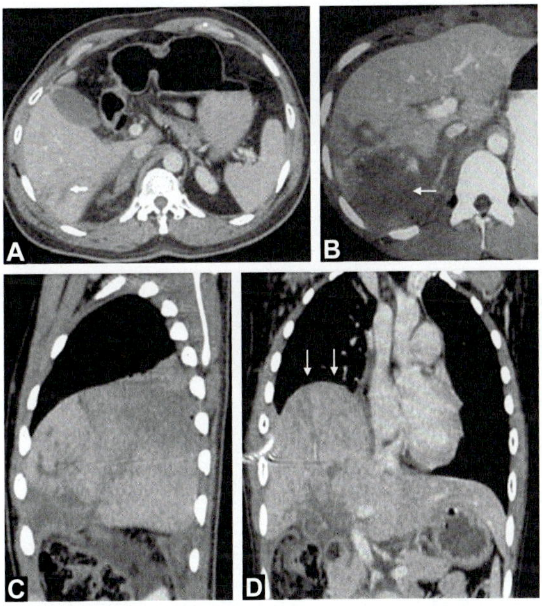


**Figs 6.4A to D:** (A) Contrast CT abdomen shows small contusions in liver; (B) Contrast CT abdomen shows lacerated liver; (C and D) CT images in a patient with diaphragmatic rupture with herniation of liver in the thorax

## HEPATIC HEMANGIOMA

Hemangioma is the most common benign tumor of the liver. The classic findings of hemangioma on CT show hyperattenuation similar to that of vessels; on dynamic contrast-enhanced CT peripheral globular enhancement and a centripetal fill in pattern with the attenuation of enhancing areas identical to that of the aorta and blood pool (Figs 6.5A to D).

On USG the need for contrast arises when the lesions are isoechoic to the background parenchyma or are diffusely isoechoic and are difficult to pick up or be characterized by B mode ultrasound. Therefore, the use of USG contrast has significantly changed the capability of ultrasound imaging. A 17-year-old male reported with general weakness, was subjected to ultrasound followed by contrast enhanced scan with SONOVUE by BRACCO (Figs 6.6A to E).

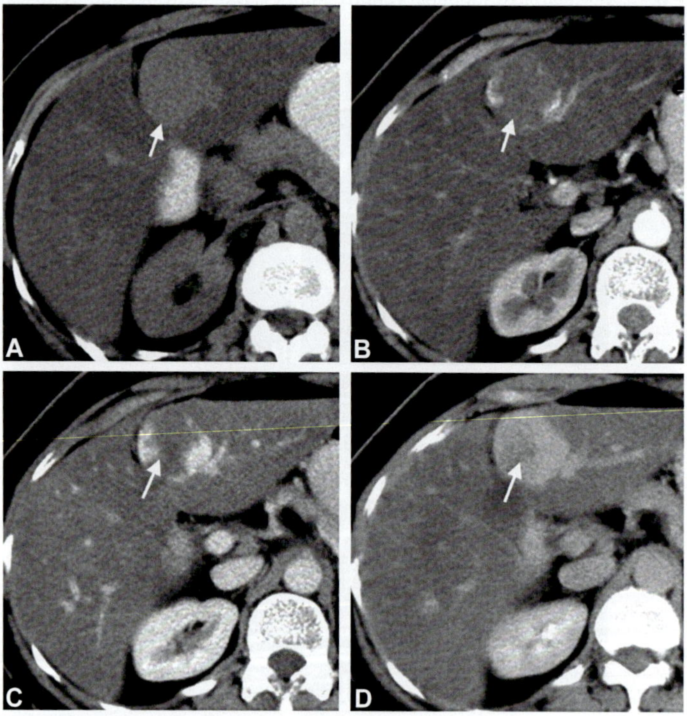


**Figs 6.5A to D:** Well-defined hyperdense lesion is seen in liver (arrow) that shows peripheral enhancement in arterial phase and progressive centripetal fill in delayed phases

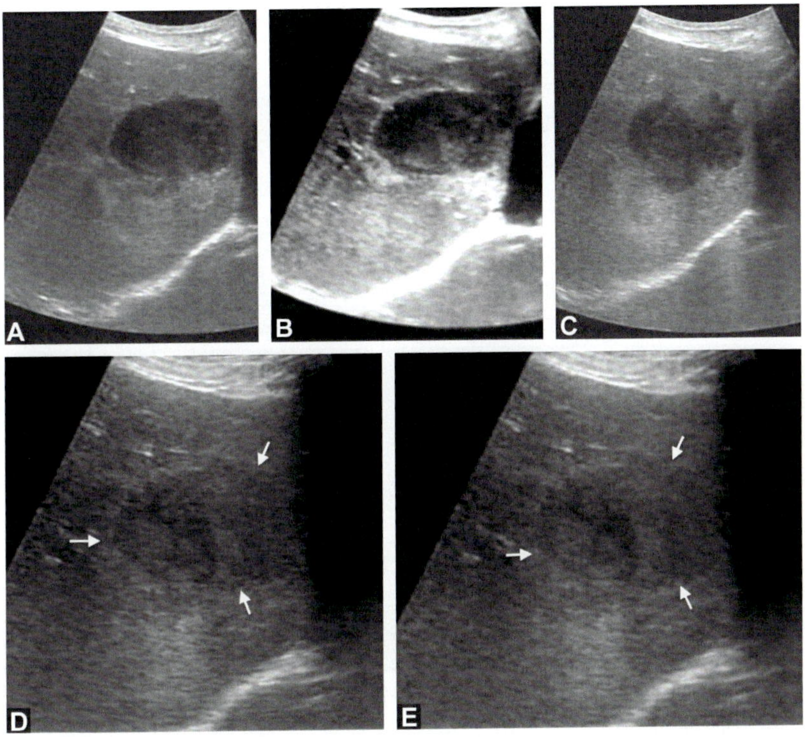


Figs 6.6A to E: (A) On ultrasound right lobe of liver shows a well-defined hypoechoic lesion; (B) Intravenous contrast injected, in arterial phase shows outlining the edges of the lesion seen as increased echogenicity of the margins of the lesion; (C) Gradually the circulating contrast shows early filling up the lesion more in the anterior aspect. As a result of peripheral filling there is some change in shape and outline of the lesion; (D and E) Show excellent filling of the lesion resulting in echogenicity isodense to the hepatic tissue which was hypoechoic in precontrast image

## HEPATOCELLULAR CARCINOMA

It is the most common primary malignant hepatic tumor.

The primary etiologic factors include hepatitis B virus and aflatoxin exposure. In areas of low incidence it occurs in old age and most patients have underlying cirrhosis caused by alcohol abuse, hemochromatosis or toxin exposure.

Symptoms are insidious in onset and include malaise, fever and abdominal pain. Jaundice may be there with elevated alpha fetoprotein.

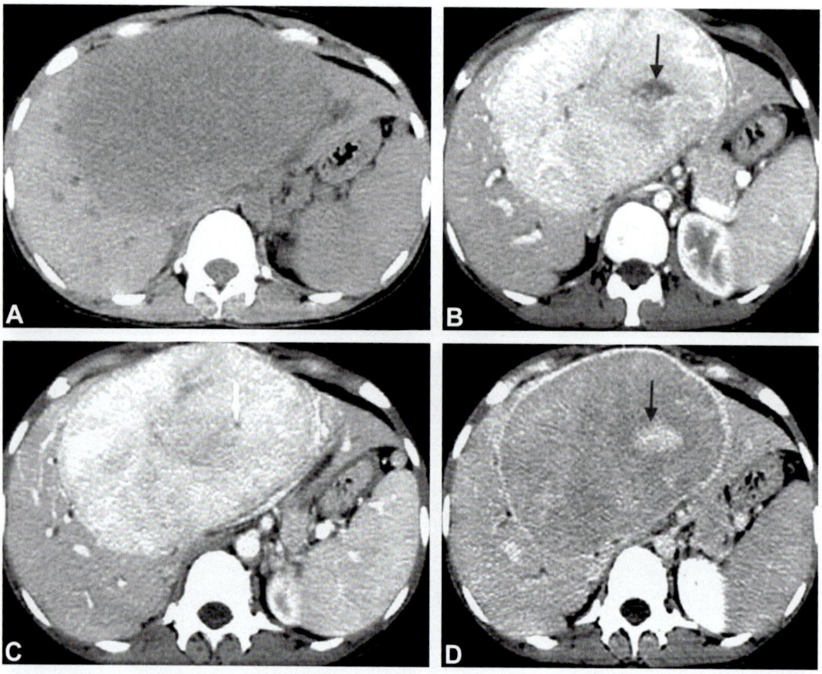

**Figs 6.7A to D:** Elderly female had right upper quadrant pain: (A) Plain CT abdomen shows mass in liver; (B) Arterial phase CT shows enhancement in the mass. A hypodense scar is also seen (arrow); (C) Venous phase CT shows enhancement in the mass as well as the scar (arrow); (D) In delayed phase CT there is persistence of contrast in the scar. This differentiates hepatocellular carcinoma from it fibronodular hyperplasia

Plain X-ray shows hepatomegaly or calcification may be seen rarely. On ultrasound it may appear as hypoechoic or hyperechoic lesion which alters the contour of the liver. Vascular invasion can be detected by Doppler examination by presence of arterial signal in thrombus.

CT demonstrates HCC as a large hypodense or isodense mass often with central areas of low attenuation representing areas of necrosis. CECT reveals enhancement of the non-necrotic areas. Vascular invasion of the portal vein, hepatic veins and IVC can also be seen (Figs 6.7A to D). CT features of portal vein invasion include arterioportal fistulas, periportal streaks of high attenuation and dilatation of main portal vein or its major branches and portal vein thrombosis.

**MR:** They reveal a variable appearance on T1WI depending on the degree of fatty change, internal fibrosis, hemorrhage and dominant histology.

**T2WI:** It appears hyperintense with necrotic areas having higher signal intensity.

**Angiography:** It demonstrates dilated feeding vessels, abundant abnormal vessels and arteriovenous shunting. Portal vein invasion produces threads and streaks appearance which is highly suggestive but not specific for HCC.

## HEPATOBLASTOMA

Hepatoblastoma is the most common primary liver tumor in children (Fig. 6.8), accounting for 79% of pediatric liver malignancies in children younger than 15 years.

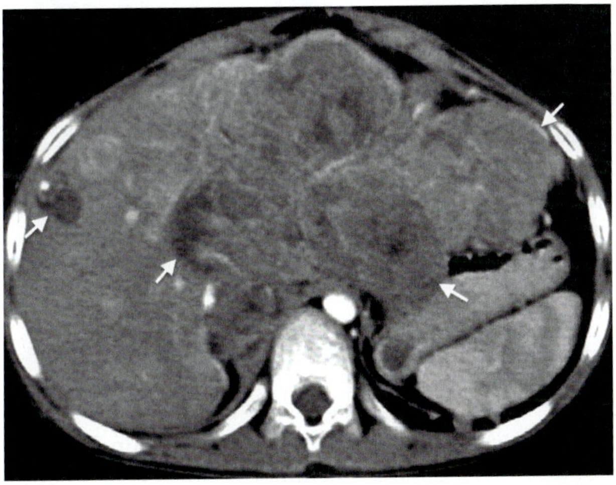

Fig. 6.8: A 12 years old male with pain in abdomen and fever since 20 days diagnosed on CT as hepatoblastoma

## HEPATIC METASTASES

Colorectal cancer, carcinoid, islet cell tumors, renal cancer, lymphoma, sarcoma, adenocarcinoma, bronchogenic carcinoma, breast, pancreas, ovarian cancer or cystadenocarcinoma can all result in hepatic metastases (Figs 6.9A to D).

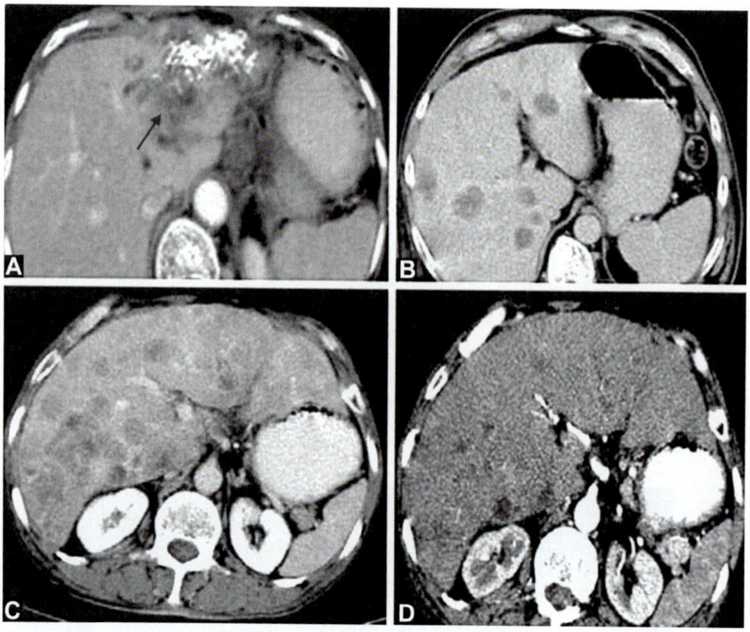


**Figs 6.9A to D:** (A) Contrast CT abdomen shows differential enhancement in the left lobe and an ill-defined low density mass which was hepatic metastases from mucinous carcinoma of transverse colon; (B to D) Enlarged liver shows multiple round hypodense metastatic lesions in both the lobes. Those of which are more hypodense in center indicate onset of necrosis

## ULTRASONOGRAPHY IN CHOLECYSTITIS (ACUTE AND CHRONIC)

### Acute Cholecystitis

Acute cholecystitis presents with acute abdominal pain. The most common cause in about 90% cases is a calculus causing cystic duct obstruction. Ultrasonography (USG) is the investigation of choice in patients with suspected acute cholecystitis, its complications and other gallbladder (GB) pathology.

Sonographic features in acute cholecystitis are presence of gallstones, distention of GB with thickening of wall due to edema with mucosal irregularity (Figs 6.10A and B). Color Doppler study shows increased vascularity in the GB wall. USG Murphy's sign is positive.

Complications of acute cholecystitis are perforation of gallbladder, pericholecystic abscess and empyema of gallbladder.

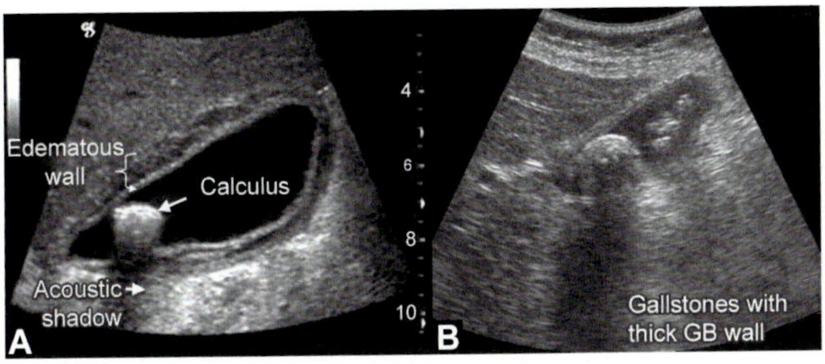


**Figs 6.10A and B:** USG gallbladder in two different cases: (A) Shows solitary GB calculus; (B) Shows multiple GB calculi. In both A and B, the calculi show acoustic shadowing, there is distention of GB with thickening of wall due to edema with mucosal irregularity

### Chronic Cholecystitis

Chronic cholecystitis is generally asymptomatic or present with mild right hypochondium pain and is associated with the presence of gallstones with or without GB wall thickning (Figs 6.11A and B). GB is not distended and Murphy's sign is absent on USG.

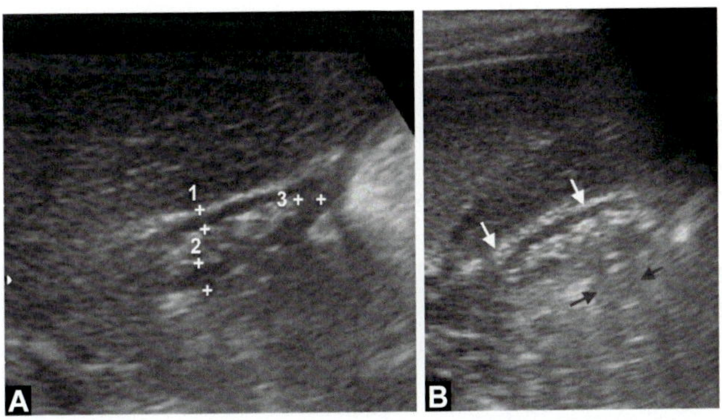


**Figs 6.11A and B:** GB is contracted and loaded with calculi obliterating the GB cavity

## CHOLELITHIASIS

Gallstone disease is common worldwide. Common risk factors for development of gallstone are obesity, diabetes, hemolytic anemia and increasing age. A common saying for risk factors is a fatty fertile female of forty years.

Most patients are asymptomatic, about 20% present with biliary colic another about 2% present with acute cholecystitis (Figs 6.10A and B).

## Composition of Gallstone or Type of Gallstones

### *Cholesterol Stone (70%)*

They can be pure cholesterol stones (not visible on plain X-rays) or may be the main component of the calculi, i.e. mixture of cholesterol + calcium carbonate/bilirubinate and are referred as mixed stones these are radiopaque on plain films and appear laminated.

### *Pigment Stone (30%)*

These are formed due to precipitation of calcium bilirubinate and contain less than 25% of cholesterol. They are usually found in association with inflammation/infection of gallbladder. On plain radiograph appear as multiple, tiny, faceted or speculated homogeneously radiopaque stones.

### *Gas Containing Gallstone*

Show radiating streak like lucency within the stone (Mercedes-Benz sign).

## GALLBLADDER IN HEPATITIS

In hepatitis gallbladder frequently shows non specific changes like thickening of gallbladder wall > 3 mm, multiple focal noncontiguous hypoechoic pockets of edema, fluid within the thickened wall may be seen (Figs 6.12A and B). Other changes can be a thin rim of fluid representing

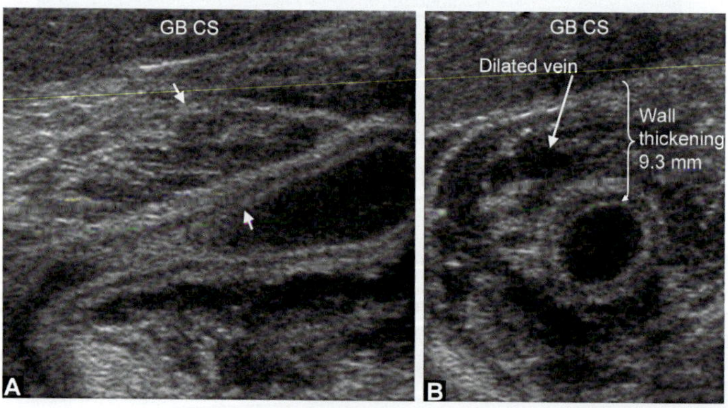


**Figs 6.12A and B:** Gallbladder shows gross thickening of the wall (between the arrows in A) due to edema and dilated veins seen within the wall (B) in a four years old child with hepatitis

edema in the wall, a double wall appearance or presence of sludge in the gallbladder cavity.

## CHOLEDOCHAL CYST

Choledochal cyst is an uncommon congenital cyst of bile duct. It usually manifest in childhood presenting with a triad of jaundice, right upper quadrant pain and palpable sub costal mass. It may be associated with cystic disease of kidney, renal tubular ectasia and medullary sponge kidney.

In Todani's choledochal cyst classification there are 5 types (Fig. 6.13) of choledochal cysts.

Type I: Fusiform cystic dilation of extrahepatic common bile duct (CBD)

Type II: Eccentric fluid filled cyst arising from CBD

Type III: Localized cystic dilation of the distal intramural duodenal portion of the CBD (choledochocele).

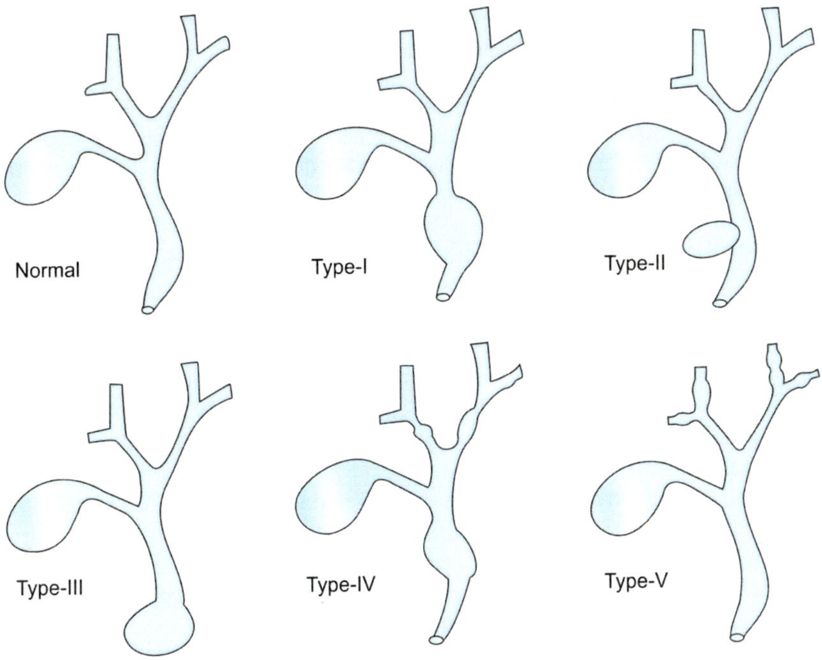


Fig. 6.13: Types of choledochal cysts

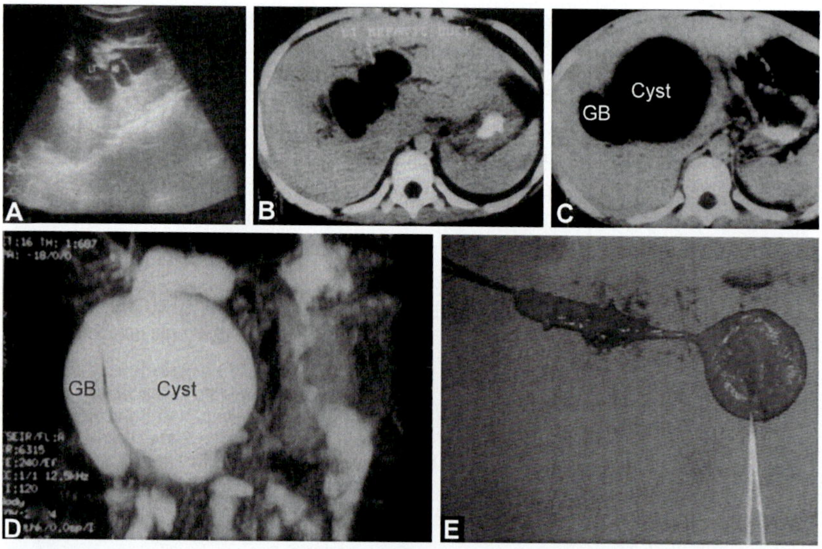


**Figs 6.14A to E:** (A) US shows the dilated, tortuous and ecstatic left hepatic duct (type IV B choledochal cyst); (B) CECT demonstrates a large cyst lying medial to gallbladder; (C) CECT shows the dilated, tortuous and ectatic left hepatic duct (similar to USG Figure A) with minimal dilatation of intrahepatic biliary radicles; (D) MRI cholangiography shows the cyst medial to the gallbladder with dilated left hepatic duct; (E) Photograph of resected specimen shows choledochal cyst, gallbladder and the cystic duct

Type IV A: Single or multiple cysts involving intra as well as extra-hepatic bile ducts

Type IV B: Single or multiple cysts involving extrahepatic bile ducts only.

Type V (Caroli's disease): Single or multiple intrahepatic bile duct cysts.

USG is the imaging modality of choice for initial evaluation. CT and MRI accurately show the location, number and extent of choledochal cyst (Figs 6.14A to E).

Endoscopic retrograde cholangiopancreaticography (ERCP) provides better appreciation of anatomical abnormality but is invasive procedure. Magnetic resonance cholangiopancreaticography (MRCP) can detect and define morphological characteristic and can detect presence of anomalous union of pancreatic and bile ducts.

Complication of choledochal cyst includes cholelithiasis, pancreatitis, biliary cirrhosis, rupture of the cyst with bile peritonitis and intrahepatic abscess and may develop biliary tract neoplasm.

## PANCREATITIS

Acute pancreatitis is an acute, diffuse inflammatory process of the pancreas that shows great variation in the degree of involvement of pancreas and the adjacent retroperitoneal tissues.

### Causes

1. Alcohol abuse, biliary tract disease, gallstones, peptic ulcer.
2. Surgery, hypotensive shock, pregnancy and trauma.
3. Hyperlipoproteinemia, hypocalcemia.
4. Drugs—azathioprine, estrogens, corticosteroids and thiazides.
5. Idiopathic fibrosing pancreatitis.
6. Infectious agents (mumps, mycoplasma, ascaris, campylobacter).

### Classification

Two major groups depending on combination of clinical, laboratory and imaging findings.

1. Mild acute pancreatitis or edematous pancreatitis occurs in 75-80% of cases. It is characterized by the parenchymal interstitial edema, absent or minimal organ dysfunction and rapid uneventful recovery without lasting consequences.
2. Severe acute pancreatitis is seen in minority of cases and is characterized by presence of parenchymal necrosis, retroperitoneal fat necrosis, systemic and distal organ failure, a protracted clinical course with lethal complication.

Initial diagnosis is based on clinical and laboratory investigation, imaging helps to authenticate clinical diagnosis and detect complications if any.

Plain X-rays, barium examination reveals secondary changes in the adjacent organs. USG, CT, MRI allows a direct visualization of pancreatic parenchyma, peripancreatic inflammation and complication.

### Complication

- Pseudopancreatic cyst
- Pseudocyst dissecting into adjacent organs
- Obstruction to bile duct
- Gastrointestinal hemorrhage due to direct erosion of blood vessel or from variceal bleed.

**Pancreatic pseudocyst** is a fluid collection that has developed a well defined nonepithelialised walls in response to extravasated enzymes (Figs 6.15A to D). It is seen in 10-20% cases. Four to six weeks are necessary for development of pseudocyst following acute pancreatitis.

### Criteria for Decompression of a Pseudocyst

- Persistence greater than 6 weeks
- Larger than 5 cm in diameter without evidence of ongoing regression
- Smaller pseudocysts causing symptoms
- Complications such as infection and internal hemorrhage.

### Treatment

a. Surgical decompression
b. Endoscopic cystogastrostomy
c. Image guided decompression
d. Percutaneous transgastric drainage is a combined technique of percutaneous gastrotomy with cystogastrostomy performed under fluoroscopy or USG guidance.

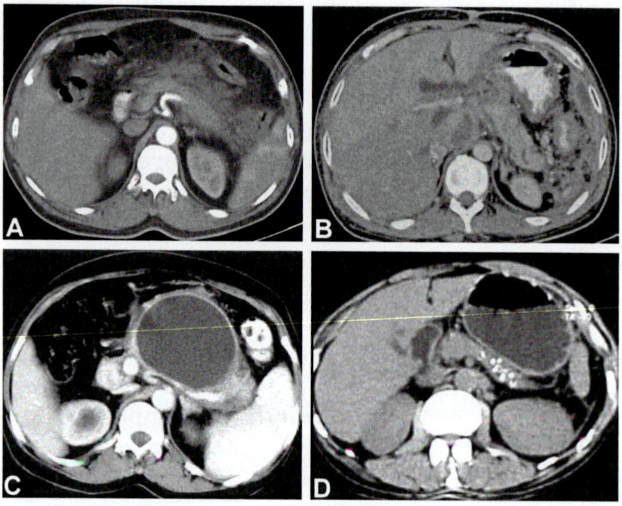

**Figs 6.15A to D:** (A) Pancreas is bulky with extensive peripancreatic fat stranding which also extends to Gerota fascia and perirenal fat; (B) Parenchymal interstitial edema presence of parenchymal necrosis, retroperitoneal fat necrosis; (C) Contrast CT abdomen shows a hypodense pseudocyst of pancreas with thick enhancing walls in the lesser sac anterior to the body and tail of pancreas which are barely perceptible; (D) Axial CT abdomen shows chronic atrophic pancreatitis with speckled to nodular calcification in the tail and body of pancreas

## SPLENUNCULUS

Splenunculus or accessory spleen is congenital nodule, composed of normal splenic tissue (Figs 6.16A and B). The spleen forms from multiple smaller components during embryogenesis, and failure of this fusion leads to one or more nodules or splenunculi remaining separate. They are extraperitoneal, benign and asymptomatic and should not be confused with splenosis which is acquired and intraperitoneal.

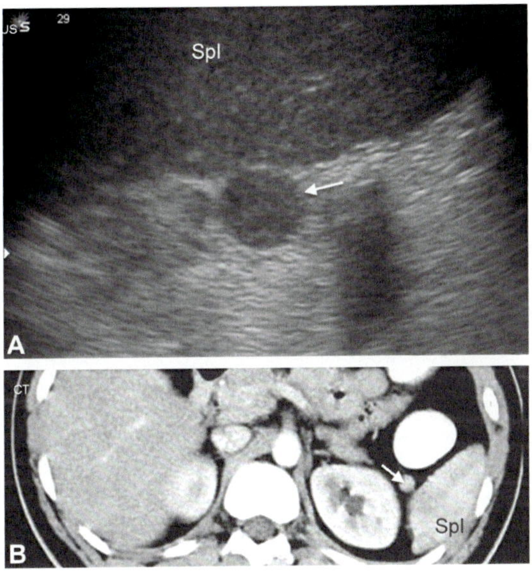


**Figs 6.16A and B:** (A) Ultrasound image shows a small round structure medial to spleen (arrow), the splenunculus. It has same echo signatures as spleen; (B) Contrast CT image shows a small round structure medial to spleen, the splenunculus (arrow). It has same density as spleen

## SPLENECTOMY

Adult spleen is convex superolaterally, concave inferomedially. It lies between the fundus of the stomach and the diaphragm, with its long axis in the line of the left tenth rib. The diaphragmatic surface is convex and is usually situated between the ninth and eleventh ribs. The visceral or inferomedial surface has gentle indentations where it comes into contact with the stomach, left kidney, pancreas, and splenic flexure. The spleen is suspended by the splenorenal ligament, the phrenicocolic and gastrosplenic ligaments. The average adult spleen measures 12 cm in length, 7 cm in breadth and 3 to 4 cm in thickness.

Spleen functions include phagocytosis, fetal hematopoiesis, adult lymphopoiesis, immune response and erythrocyte storage.

Indications of elective splenectomy are:

1. Symptomatic massive splenomegaly.
2. Certain cases of wandering spleen.
3. Idiopathic thrombocytopenic purpura.
4. Post-traumatic splenic hematoma/laceration.
5. Following spontaneous rupture.
6. For long-term treatment of congenital erythropoietic porphyria.
7. For diagnosing certain lymphomas.
8. The spread of gastric cancer to splenic tissue.

### *Complications of splenectomy are:*

- Sepsis (such as *Streptococcus pneumoniae* and *Haemophilus influenzae*)
- Leukocytosis (increase in blood leukocytes)
- Thrombocytosis (increase in blood platelet count) can lead to an increased risk of potentially fatal clot formation.

CHAPTER

# 7 Urogenital System

**Chapter Outline**



## INTRAVENOUS UROGRAPHY

Intravenous urogram (IVU) is the radiology procedure to visualize the excretory function of kidney, pelvicalyceal system, ureters and urinary bladder after injecting 40 to 60 ml of intravenous contrast (Fig. 7.1).

### Indications for IVU

1. Congenital anomalies
   a. Horseshoe kidney
   b. Duplex kidney and double ureters
   c. Polycystic kidney disease

    d. Retrocaval ureter
    e. Ureterocele.
2. Hydronephrosis
3. To ascess renal function
4. Renal injury
5. Renal tumors
6. Postsurgery for urinary leak, fistulae and stricture.

### Contraindications for IVU

1. Iodine sensitivity
2. Multiple myeloma
3. Hypergammaglobulinemias.
   Precaution should be taken in patients with diabetes, hypertension and dehydration.

### Procedural Requirement Include

1. Overnight fasting for 8 hours
2. Bowel preparation with laxatives to reduce abdominal gases
3. Renal function tests to ascertain serum creatinine and blood urea levels are within normal limits indicating that renal function is not impaired.

### Procedure

1. First, a plain X-ray KUB is taken and then 0.5 ml test dose of sodium diatrizoate (urografin) or meglumine iothalamate is injected IV and wait for 5 minutes for any reaction. If no adverse reaction occurs, then full, dose, i.e. one ml/kg body weight, IV urografin is given (40-60 ml). However, today contrast media are very safe.
2. X-ray KUB is taken after 3 to 5 minutes, which shows the nephrographic and secretory function of the kidneys.
3. Followed by 15 minutes and then 20 to 30 minutes films are taken.
4. Further films are taken depending on the requrement of the specific case. Delayed films up to 72 hours are occasionally indicated.
5. In case of renal failure with high serum creatinine and blood urea levels IVU is avoided and patient should be subjected to alternative imaging protocol.
6. Abdominal compression is done to have better definition of calyces, but not done in children and patients with abdominal aortic aneurysm.

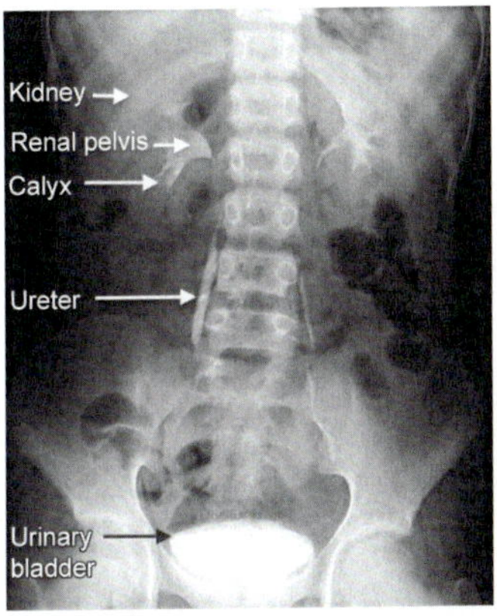


**Fig. 7.1:** Normal intravenous urogram

## DUPLICATION OF URETER

The duplication of ureter may be incomplete (the ureters fusing at some point in their course and having a common distal orifices) or complete (both ureters having separate distal orifices). Incomplete duplication is almost always of no clinical significance. It may be bilateral (Figs 7.2A and B) or unilateral (Figs 7.3A to G). Although in a small proportion of cases it may

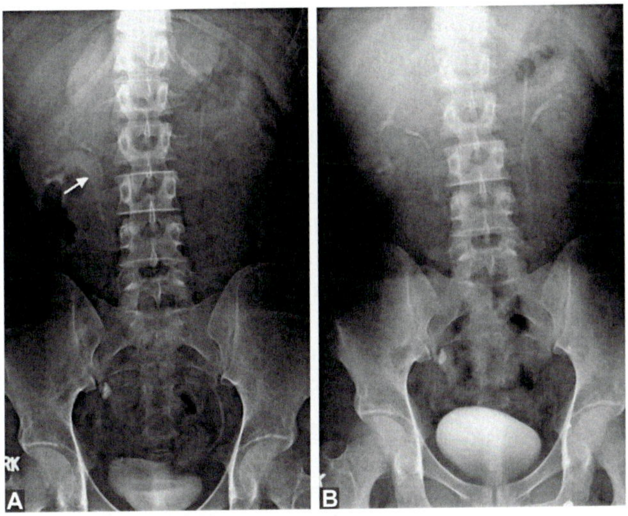


**Figs 7.2A and B:** IVP X-rays shows incomplete bilateral duplication of ureters. On right side lower moiety has extrarenal pelvis. Calcified gland is seen close to inferior aspect of right SI joint

be associated with yo-yo reflux in which urine from one ureter refluxes back up the other ureter. This may lead to loin pain on micturition and urinary tract infection.

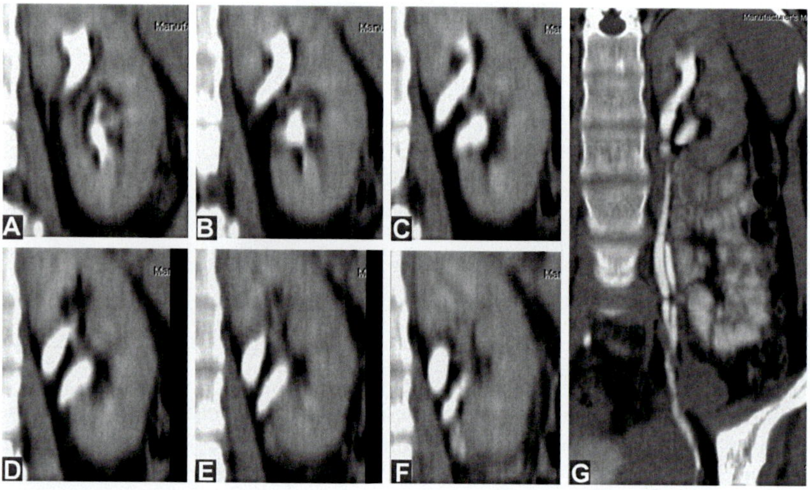

**Figs 7.3A to G:** Intravenous urogram shows left kidney (A to C) two pelvicalyceal collecting systems, twin pelvis and ureter seen in D to F. G is coronal reconstruction, shows left kidney with twin collecting system and two ureters which unite at L4 level

## HORSESHOE KIDNEY

Horseshoe kidney is most frequent developmental anomaly where there is failure of complete ascent of kidneys with the fusion of lower poles across the midline by the isthmus lying anterior or posterior to the aorta and inferior vena cava. It is due to fusion of subdivisions of mesonephric duct, when the embryo is 30 to 40 days old preventing ascent of kidney. The kidney is always ectopic and lies lower than the normal. The commonest site is in front of forth lumbar vertebra.

Horseshoe kidney presents as a fixed, nonmobile, firm mass in the midline at the level of 4th lumbar vertebra which is resonant on percussion. It is prone to infection, stone formation, hydronephrosis and trauma.

### Diagnosis

1. On plain X-ray abdomen one may infrequently be able to appreciate the outline of the horseshoe kidney.

2. On IVU kidneys are lower than normal in position and are oriented vertically close to spine. Ureter curves laterally and then assumes a normal medial course like a 'flower vase' (Figs 7.4A to C).
3. USG abdomen helps to detect associated complications like calculus or hydronephrosis.

It may be associated with anomalies like PUJ obstruction, duplex collecting system or ureterocele. It may be associated with Turner's syndrome or trisomy 13.

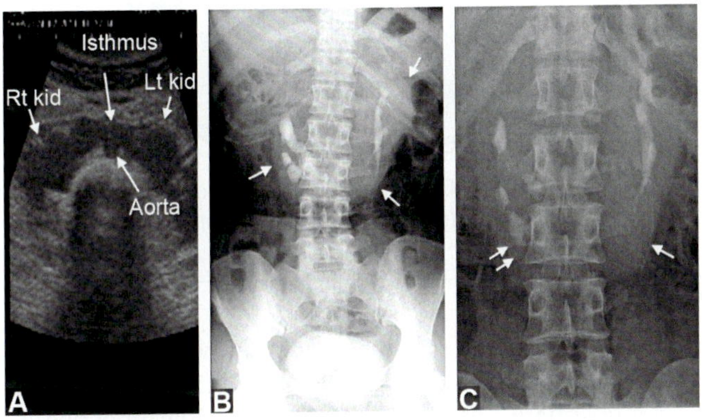


**Figs 7.4A to C:** (A) USG shows horseshoe kidneys with the fusion of lower poles across the midline by the isthmus lying anterior to the aorta; (B) and (C) on IVU kidneys (arrows in B) are lower than normal in position and are oriented vertically close to spine, the ureter curves laterally and then assumes a normal medial course (arrows in C) like a 'flower vase'

## LEFT RENAL APLASIA

Renal aplasia is the predominant cause of congenital solitary kidneys (Figs 7.5A and B). Congenital solitary kidneys, which are susceptible to renal failure, have been considered mostly due to unilateral renal agenesis and partly due to renal aplasia. Risk of familial recurrence and of other associated anomalies is known to be much higher in renal agenesis than in renal aplasia. However, differential diagnosis between the two renal anomalies is difficult, and renal agenesis has been found much less frequently in ultrasound screening studies of fetuses than in autopsy studies.

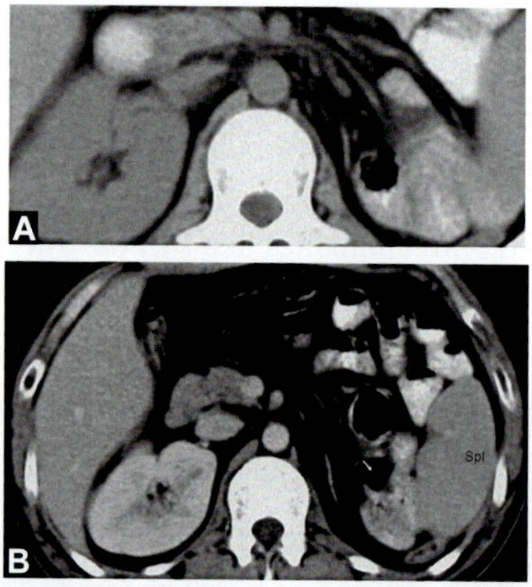


**Figs 7.5A and B:** (A) Plain; (B) Contrast CT images show absence of left kidney. The left renal fossa is occupied by intestinal loops

## STAGHORN CALCULUS

Staghorn calculus is a smooth surfaced calculus occupying the renal pelvis and calyces. It is composed of phosphate or calcium and ammonium magnesium phosphate hence also known as triple phosphate calculus. It may be unilateral or bilateral with possibly pre-existing infection with proteolytic organism like proteus or *E.coli*. The clinical triad of presentation is mass, fever and hematuria.

Complications of staghorn calculus are pyelonephritis, pyonephrosis, perinephric abscess and renal failure.

Plain X-ray abdomen for kidney, ureter and bladder (KUB) area shows a large radio dense calculus in the renal fossa depending on the size adopts the pevicalyceal shape (Fig. 7.6). Ultrasonography abdomen shows a hyperechoic calculus in the renal pelvis and calyceal system with hydronephrosis or any associated complication. Intravenous urogram (IVU) shows the renal function.

Under antibiotic cover percutaneous nephrolithotomy (PCNL) is becoming a popular procedure for staghorn calculi. In cases of unilateral calculus nephropyelolithotomy is performed. In bilateral disease the kidney which is functioning better should be treated first and after three months or later the other kidney is operated upon.

In bilateral staghorn calculi with pyonephrosis, bilateral nephrostomy is done using Malecott catheter (Cabot's nephrostomy). If function is present, then both kidneys are operated one after the other with a suitable gap.

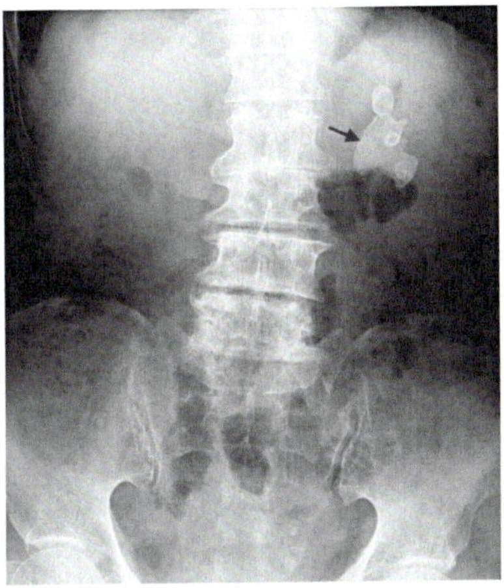

Fig. 7.6: Plain X-ray KUB shows staghorn calculus (arrow) on left side

## MULTICYSTIC DYSPLASTIC KIDNEY DISEASE

High resolution ultrasonography allows demonstration of fetal kidneys and urinary bladder from second trimester and enables to detect major congenital anomalies of the urinary system (Figs 7.7A to C). Multicystic dysplastic kidney disease (MCDKD) is usually an incidental finding during routine antenatal sonographic examination. The incidence of MCDKD is about 1 in 10,000 births.

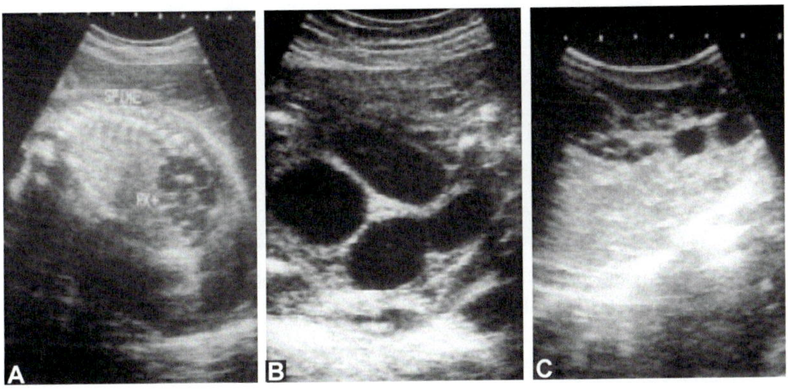


Figs 7.7A to C: (A) Antenatal ultrasound shows enlarged right fetal kidney with multiple cysts; (B) and (C) Postabortion ultrasound shows enlarged kidneys with multiple cysts

## POLYCYSTIC KIDNEY DISEASE

Polycystic kidney disease (PKD) is an autosomal dominant trait and is much more common in adults. An autosomal recessive form of PKD also exists and appears in infancy or childhood. In early stages of the disease, the cysts cause the kidney to swell up (Figs 7.8A and B), disrupting kidney function and leading to chronic high blood pressure and kidney infections. Bleeding in a cyst can cause flank pain. Kidney stones are more common in PKD. PKD may be associated with brain aneurysms, cysts in the liver, pancreas, and testes and colonic diverticula.

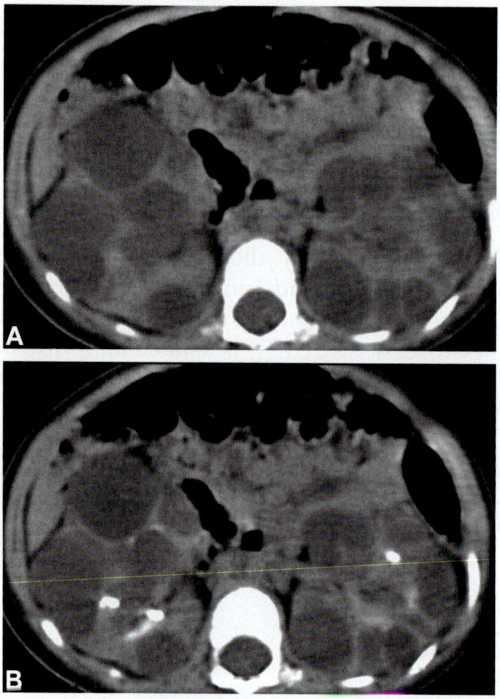


**Figs 7.8A and B:** Plain and contrast CT abdomen shows bilateral polycystic kidneys with parenchymal thinning and delayed excretion of contrast

## OBSTRUCTIVE UROPATHY

Obstructive uropathy results in hydronephrosis and hydroureter depending on the site of mechanical obstruction. Hydronephrosis is dilation of the calyces and renal pelvis appearing on ultrasound as anechoic areas and gradually there is reduction in renal cortical thickness (Figs 7.9A and B). Ultrasound is a quick, safe and sensitive tool for detecting hydronephrosis and possibly the cause.

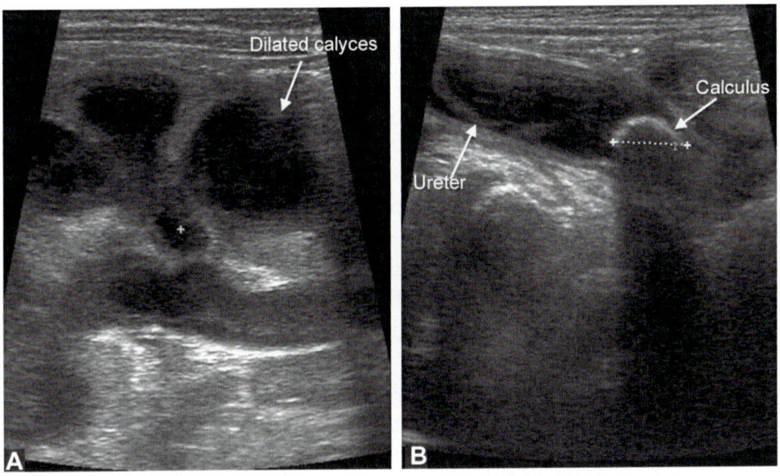


**Figs 7.9A and B:** (A) 9 mm diameter calculus is seen in proximal ureter; (B) with acoustic shadowing and resultant hydronephrosis and hydroureter (A and B) with marked thinning of renal cortex. There is thickening of wall of ureter with internal echos in dilated ureter are suggestive of inflammatory process

## Unilateral Hydronephrosis

Hydronephrosis is an aseptic dilation of pelvicalyceal system (Figs 7.10A to C) due to partial or intermittent obstruction to the outflow of urine.

Causes of unilateral hydronephrosis are:

a. *Intraluminal:* Renal pelvic or ureteric calculus and sloughed papilla.
b. *Intramural:* Pelviureteric obstruction, ureterocele or ureteric stricture due to tuberculosis, post-traumatic, endometriosis, radiation fibrosis or ureteral tumors.
c. *Extramural:* Aberrant renal artery or vein, extrinsic compression by growth or retroperitoneal fibrosis.

## Pelviureteric Junction Obstruction

Idiopathic obstruction at the pelviureteric junction (PUJ) is major cause of obstructive uropathy at all ages and is the most common cause of neonatal hydronephrosis. More than half the cases, obstruction is functional due to deficiency of muscle fibers with an increase in collagen tissue. This results in an impaired transmission of the peristaltic waves from the renal pelvis to the ureter (segmental dysfunction or adynamic segment). Other causes are intrinsic stenosis of the PUJ are due to infolding of the local mucosa and musculature or local kink and angulation of the ureter associated with adhesions and overlying fibrous bands. An aberrant renal artery to the lower pole of the kidney may result in PUJ obstruction. It may occur in a duplex system where it almost always affects the lower moiety. Malrotated, horseshoe kidney and ectopic kidneys are prone to PUJ obstruction.

PUJ obstruction occurs more commonly in males than females and is more frequent on left side. There can be bilateral involvement in 10 to 30 % of patients. Newborns and infants present with a palpable abdominal lump. Older children may present with intermittent abdominal pain with vomiting, hematuria or urinary tract infection.

USG shows hydronephrosis with dilated calyces and associated cortical atrophy. On intravenous urography (IVU) delayed opacification of the collecting system, pyelocaliectasis, narrowing at PUJ and retention of contrast material in the collecting system on delayed films is seen. Radionuclide studies give the best objective assessment of renal function.

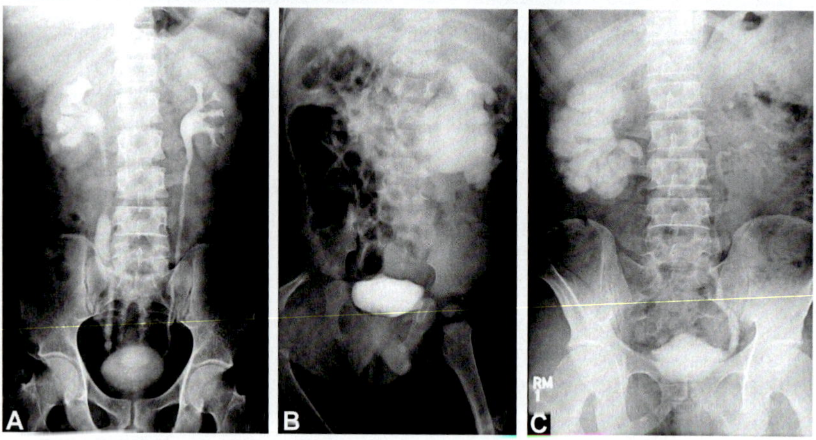


**Figs 7.10A to C:** Three different case on IVU show unilateral hydronephrosis

## Complications

a. Pyonephrosis
b. Perinephric abscess
c. Renal failure in bilateral renal involvement.

### Treatment

a. Anderson-Hyne's operation (pyeloplasty) in which the spasmodic segment and redundant pelvis are excised. A new pelvis is created and the cut end of pelvis is anastomosed to the ureter in the dependent position.
b. Davis T-tube ureterostomy is placement of T-tube in the ureter by making longitudinal incision.
c. Non-dismembered pyeloplasty is reconstruction done by Foley's Y-V plasty without PUJ transaction.

## RETROCAVAL URETER

Retrocaval ureter (Figs 7.11A and B) is a congenital anomaly. Common presentations are right lumbar pain, dull aching or intermittent (renal colic), recurrent urinary tract infections and microscopic or gross hematuria. There is a high incidence of calculi due to stasis. Diagnosis is confirmed by ultrasonography and intravenous urography. Spiral CT scan and MRI help sometimes to delineate the anatomy clearly and non-invasively.

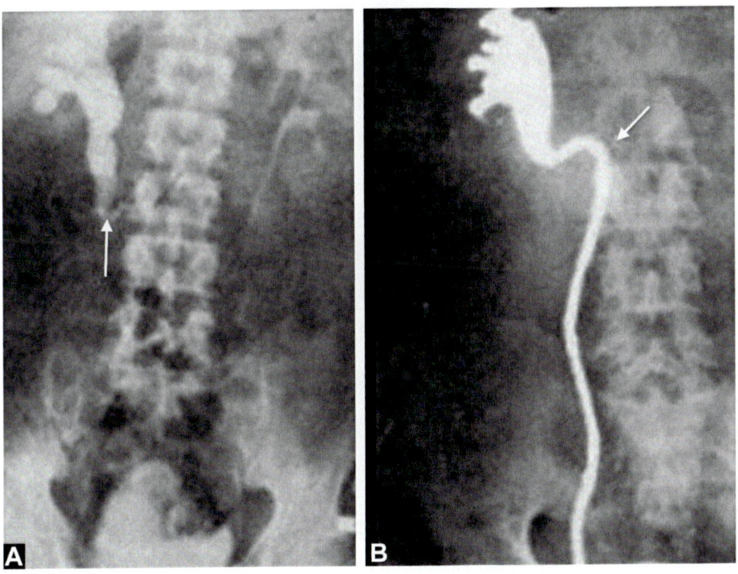


**Figs 7.11A and B:** (A) IVP shows dilated right upper ureter, and upper third ureter shows S-shaped curvature towards the midline; (B) RGP shows upper third of right ureter curving towards the midline (arrow)

## URETEROCELE

Ureterocele develops due to congenital stenosis of the ureteral orifice with resultant weakness of the wall of the lower ureter which leads to ballooning of the terminal ureter into the bladder. This intracystic ballooning of the dilated ureter produces a characteristic defect on the cystogram, which is practically pathognomonic. The size of the ureterocele may vary from a centimeter in diameter to a large size which may fill the bladder.

The obstruction is secondary to the ureterocele, so there may be frequently associated hydronephrosis on the affected side. It is commonly associated with double ureter, in such cases the ureterocele usually affects the ureter draining the upper renal moiety. Ureteroceles may also contain calculi.

On retrograde cystogram ureterocele appears as a round, constant filling defect at the ureteral orifice. On intravenous urography, the thickness of the ureterocele wall will form a non-opaque halo or cobra head appearance with contrast in the ureter, ureterocele, and bladder. If calculi are present they lie within this halo (Figs 7.12A and B).

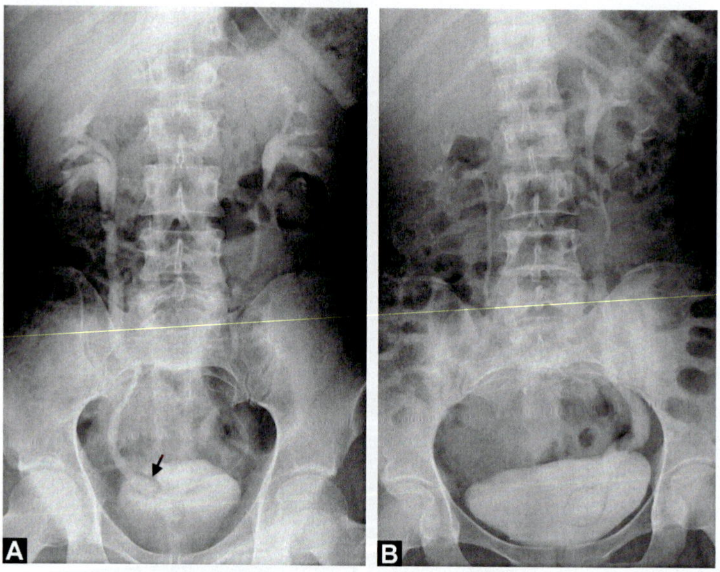


**Figs 7.12A and B:** (A) IVP study shows duplication of pelvicalyceal system on right. In the terminal part right ureter ureterocele (arrow) is present (Cobra head appearance); (B) In another case IVP study shows duplication of pelvicalyceal system on left side with ureterocele left which is draining the upper renal moiety which shows early obstructive uropathy

## MÜLLERIAN DUCT CYST

Müllerian duct cyst is an uncommon congenital anomaly. It is usually small, asymptomatic, midline, cystic lesion, located behind the superior half of the prostatic urethra and connected to the verumontanum by a thin stalk. Rarely a müllerian duct cyst may be associated with renal agenesis and hypospadias. MRI accurately defines anatomic relationship when one is planning to excise a Müllerian duct cyst (Figs 7.13A to F). Multiplanar imaging provides superior soft tissue contrast, and absence of ionizing radiation.

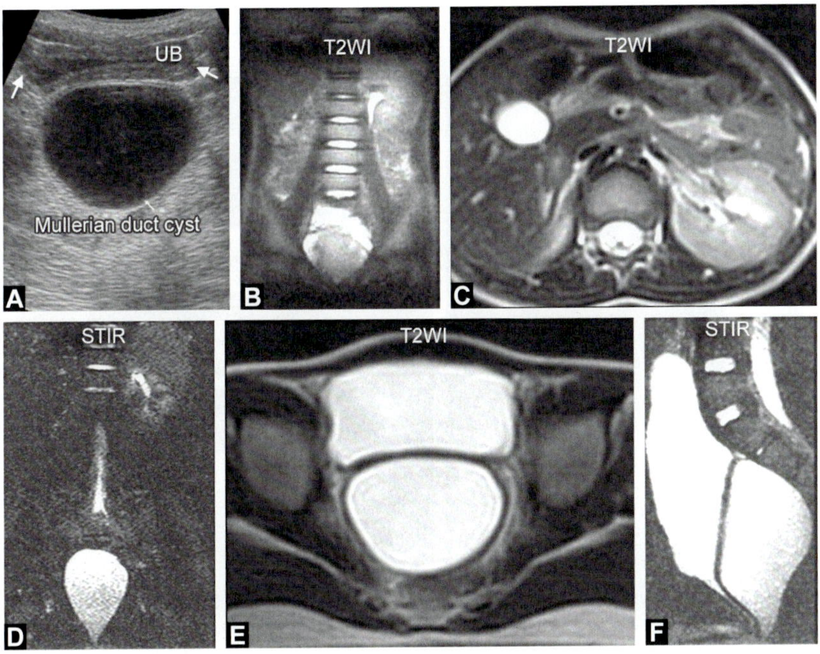


**Figs 7.13A to F:** In a 5-year-old male child transabdominal USG: (A) show cystic nature lesion posterior to bladder (arrows); (B and C) Agenesis of right kidney with normal left kidney is seen in coronal and axial T2 weighted images; (D and E) Pear shaped cystic nature mass lesion seen hyperintense on STIR and T2 weighted images; (F)Sagittal STIR MR image show that there is no communication between cystic lesion and urinary bladder

## BLADDER DIVERTICULA

Ectopia vesicae or exstrophy of bladder is a congenital abnormality in which there is incomplete development or absence of the infraumbilical part of the anterior abdominal wall, associated with incomplete development of the bladder. These cases often develop bladder diverticulae which are localized out-pouchings of the bladder mucosa (Figs 7.14A to D) between fibers of the detrusor muscles (pseudo-diverticulae) resulting from a congential or acquired defect in the bladder wall. A wide neck diverticulum fills and empties readily with the bladder, but in a narrow neck diverticulum there is poor emptying, the diverticulum may be better appreciated on postvoid film.

Renal calculus disease is relatively uncommon in children. The etiology of renal calculi in children could be due to infection, developmental anomalies of the genitourinary tract, metabolic disorders. Non-contrast CT shows virtually all stones as high attenuation foci.

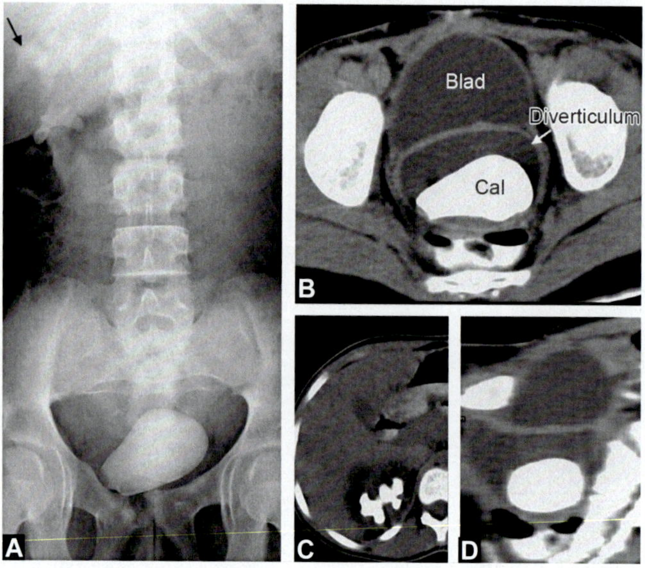


**Figs 7.14A to D:** (A) Plain X-ray abdomen shows multiple staghorn calculi in right kidney and a large calculus in bladder area; (B) CT scan demonstrates a large posterior bladder diverticulum with a large calculus; (C) The large stag horn calculus in right kidney; (D) Sagittal recon CT image shows a posterior diverticulum filled with urine and a large calculus within it

## POSTERIOR URETHRAL VALVES WITH CYSTITIS

Cystitis in children, frequently results in upper urinary tract infection (UTI) which is most often due to bacterial infection. Difference between lower UTI (cystitis) and upper UTI (pyelonephritis) is difficult in small children and rarely crucial. Imaging algorithm will be similar in both situations, an important aspect being to exclude outflow obstruction and presence of vesicoureteric reflux.

Posterior urethral valves are the frequent cause of urethral obstruction in male children. These valves are positioned at the proximal urethra the distal most portion of prostatic urethra resulting in obstruction in the flow of urine. The consequence is dilatation of prostatic urethra. The diagnostic study is micturating cystourethrogram (MCU), which should be carried out once infection is treated. MCU demonstrates dilated prostatic urethra and is treated by cystoscopic valve fulguration (Fig. 7.15).

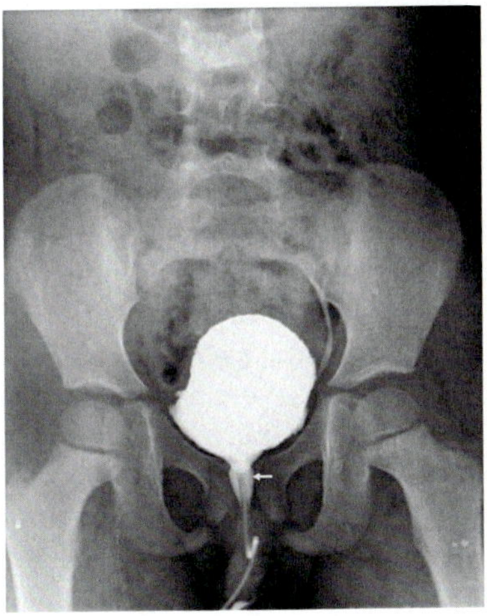

**Fig. 7.15:** Micturating cystourethrogram shows dilatation of prostatic urethra secondary to posterior urethral valves with cystitis seen as irregularity of bladder wall

## HYDROCELE

It is an abnormal collection of serous fluid between the layers of tunica vaginalis. It is a common cause of painless scrotal swelling. It can be congenital or acquired. On ultrasound hydroceles appear as anechoic collections with good acoustic transmission surrounding the anterolateral aspects of the testes (Fig. 7.16). Low level to medium level echoes from fibrin bodies or cholesterol crystal may be found within the hydroceles. Large hydrocele may impede testicular venous drainage and cause absence of antegrade arterial diastolic flow.

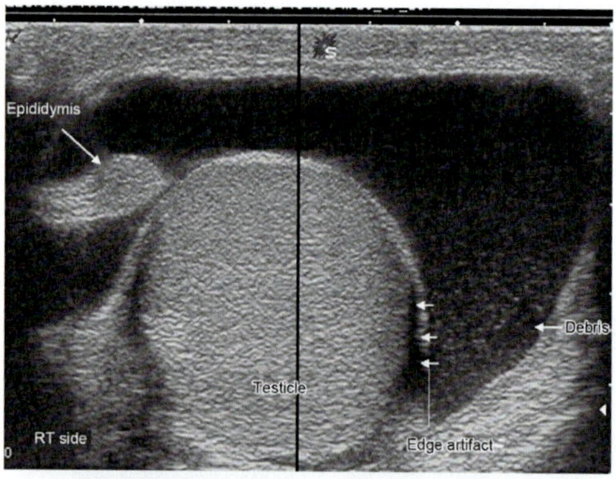


Fig. 7.16: USG shows fluid in right tunica vaginalis with internal echos indicating debris

## UNDESCENDED TESTICLE (CRYPTORCHIDISM)

If the testicle cannot be located within the scrotum, it is undescended. An undescended testicle most commonly lies in the inguinal canal or it may lie higher up along the normal line of descent in the abdominal.

If testicles fail to descend by the age of 3 years, it is associated with abnormal development and this is severe at puberty as a result undescended testes may be atrophic with poor spermatogenesis.

Ultrasound is regarded as the initial investigation to locate an undescended testicle (Figs 7.17A to C). If not identified on ultrasound, a more extensive search is desired by MRI. CT should be avoided because of radiations. On MR testicle shows a high signal on T2-weighted and STIR sequences.

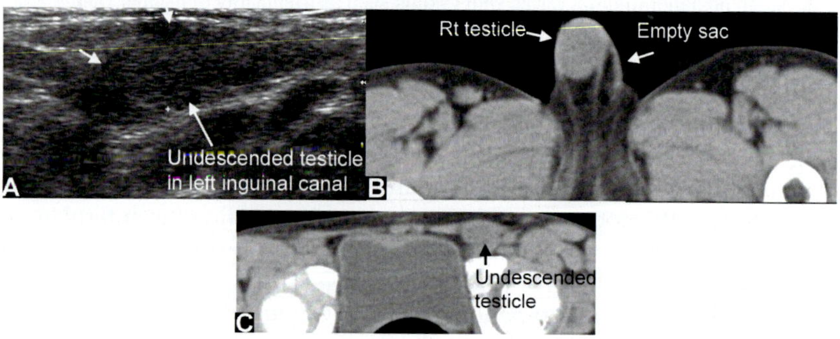


Figs 7.17A to C: (A) Left inguinal USG in oblique plane shows the undescended testicle in the inguinal canal (arrows); (B) Axial CT image shows right testicle in scrotal sac which is empty on left side; (C) Axial CT image shows undescended testicle in the left inguinal canal

## EXTRACORPOREAL SHOCK-WAVE LITHOTRIPSY

Extracorporeal shock-wave lithotripsy (ESWL) is noninvasive technique for management of the calculus by fragmenting them. Calculus is localized under fluoroscopic or ultrasound guidance. Piezoceramic or electromagnetic shock waves are passed to create compressive waves over the calculus through water bath or water cushion which acts as a media. Shocks are produced at the rate 2/sec; 1000-4000 shocks are required for each calculus. Dornier lithotripter is used for fragmenting stones followed by flushing out of these fragments.

### Advantages

1. No need of anesthesia.
2. Performed as an OPD procedure.
3. Less than 2.5 cm sized stones are well fragmented.
4. Hard stones, i.e. oxalate stones are better eliminated by ESWL.
5. ESWL can be repeated.

### Complications

a. Renal hematoma
b. Severe hematuria
c. Injury to adjacent structures
d. Fragmented stone gets lodged in the ureter.

### Contraindications

a. Pregnancy
b. Bleeding disorders
c. Patients with abdominal aneurysm
d. Sepsis and renal failure.

## WILM'S TUMOR

Wilm's tumor is the most common renal malignancy between 1 to 5 years of age with a peak at 3 years and is rare after 6 years of age. It starts from primitive undifferentiated embryonal metanephric blast cells. Most Wilm's tumors can be cured.

Clinically present as a painless palpable abdominal lump which is noticed incidentally by the parents. Fever, malaise, anorexia, hypertention, leukocytosis and gross or microscopic hematuria may occur. Other associated abnormalities like cryptorchidism, hypospadias, ambiguous genitalia, horseshoe kidney may be present. Some tumors are present in association with Beckwith-Wiedemann syndrome (BWS), bloom syndrome and trisomy 18.

Plain abdomen X-ray shows presence of mass in the flank. Ten percent or less of cases show calcification within the mass. USG is the first imaging modality of choice for detecting the tumor itself and its vascular extension. Abdominal CT is more sensitive in identifying tumor extent, vessel involvement and metastasis (Figs 7.18A to D).

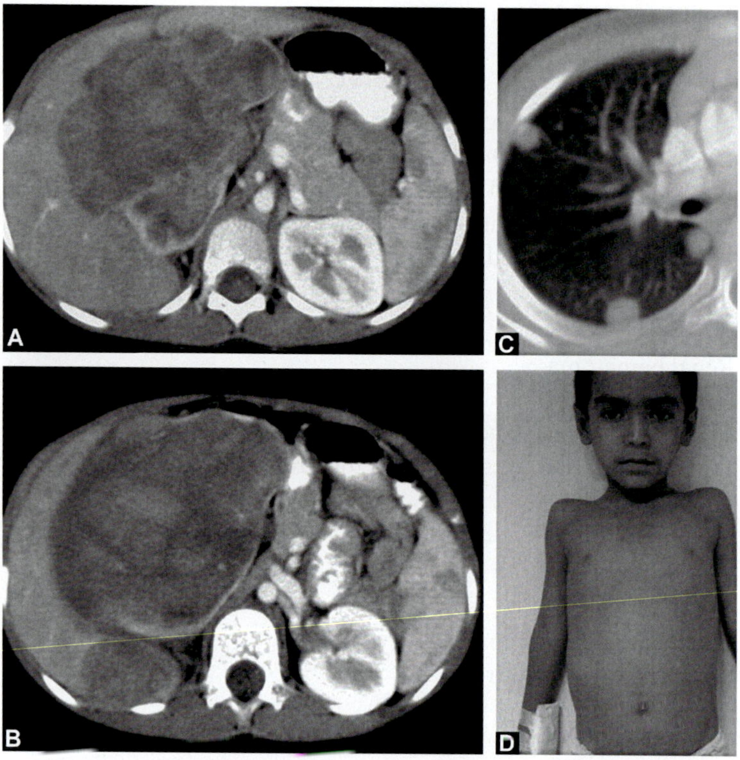

**Figs 7.18A to D:** (A) CECT shows large well defined enhancing mass lesion 9 × 10 cm with few areas of necrosis, involving the right kidney, sparing its upper pole. Medially the lesion is seen to displace the pancreas and great vessels to left side with compression of IVC. Cranially the lesion is seen to abut the inferior surface of liver and inferiorly extent to iliac crest; (B) Another 3 × 2.4 cm heterogeneously enhancing lesion is noted in posteroinferior segment of right lobe of liver is metastasis. Filling defect is noted in right renal vein which is stretched out and compression of IVC possibly tumor thrombosis; (C) Multiple well defined metastatic lesions are seen in the lungs seen in a 6 years old male child; (D) Presented with gradually increasing lump in abdomen

### Staging

1. Disease confined to kidney and is completely resectable.
2. Tumor extends beyond the kidney, but can be excised completely.
3. Residual disease after resection with positive lymph nodes and massive spillage.
4. Blood born metastasis.
5. Bilateral disease.

Prognosis depends on age, size, bilaterality of the tumor, hematuria, spread and histology of tumor.

### Treatment

1. Nephrectomy and postoperative radiotherapy in case of unilateral tumors.
2. In bilateral tumors, either bilateral partial nephrectomy or nephrectomy on one side with partial nephrectomy on the other side.
3. Followed by chemotherapy with actinomycin D, vincristine and doxorubicin.

## RENAL CELL CARCINOMA OR GRAWITZ TUMOR

Renal cell carcinoma is an adenocarcinoma arising from renal tubular cells (Fig. 7.19); most common site is proximal renal tubule. It is also known as hypernephroma a misnomer, Grawitz tumor or clear cell carcinoma. It occurs more commonly in males usually in 5th and 6th decade of life. M:F ratio is 2:1.

### Predisposing Factors

1. High animal fat in diet
2. Environmental factors like asbestos, lead, cadmium and tobacco
3. Cigarette smoking
4. Chromosomal aberration
5. Acquired cystic kidney disease after long-term dialysis
6. Association with von Hippel-Lindau (VHL) disease.

Patient usually presents with hematuria, dragging sensation in the loin, mass in the loin. Left sided varicocele may develop due to extension of the tumor thrombus into left gonadal vein.

## Spread

1. Local spread to involve perinephric pad of fat, calyces and renal pelvis.
2. RCC enters the renal vein as proliferating tumor thrombus, which extends into the IVC and right atrium, left testicular vein may also be involved.
3. Lymphatic spread takes place to hilar lymph nodes and para-aortic lymph nodes.
4. Metastases generally spreads to lung, liver, brain and bone.

## Investigations

1. Urine for RBCs.
2. IVU shows mass lesion and irregular filling defect.
3. USG abdomen to know the size and extension of the mass.
4. CT scan to confirm the diagnosis and also helps to know status of renal vein and IVC, lymph node involvement and spread to the liver.
5. Renal angiogram shows the vascularity of the tumor.
6. Chest X-ray may show cannon ball secondaries.

## Treatment

1. Surgery is the treatment of choice in the form of radical nephrectomy, nephron sparing surgery is done in bilateral RCC. Preoperative renal artery embolization is done to reduce the tumor vascularity.
2. Chemotherapy.

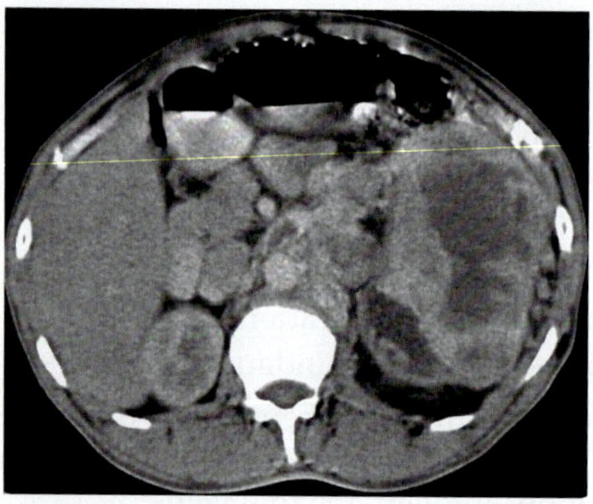

**Fig. 7.19:** Contrast enhanced CT (CECT). Shows heterogeneously enhancing mass lesion (arrows) arising from anterior cortex of left kidney. It is seen extending into left renal vein with thrombosis of the renal vein (block arrow) with enlarged nodes at renal hilum

# 8

# CHAPTER

# Obstetrics and Gynecology

Chapter Outline



## HYSTEROSALPINGOGRAM

Hysterosalpingogram (HSG) is radiological procedure of visualization of the inside of the uterus and fallopian tubes. Normal HSG demonstrates the normal anatomy of uterus and fallopian tubes with bilateral peritoneal spill (Fig. 8.1). It is ideally performed between 7th to 12th day of menstrual cycle. It may reveal abnormality of the uterus, tubal block (Figs 8.2 and 8.3) or hydrosalpinx (Fig. 8.4). If sterilization reversal is planned, the point at which the tubes are blocked can be seen (Fig. 8.5).

In this procedure, the contrast is passed through the cervix into the uterus and through the tubes into the peritoneal cavity if the tubes are not blocked by scar tissue or adhesions. Hysterosalpingography is indicated in sterility to see the patency of tubes. On HSG uterine cavity is also evaluated for the presence of congenital uterine anomalies, polyps, fibroid, tumors or uterine scar tissue.

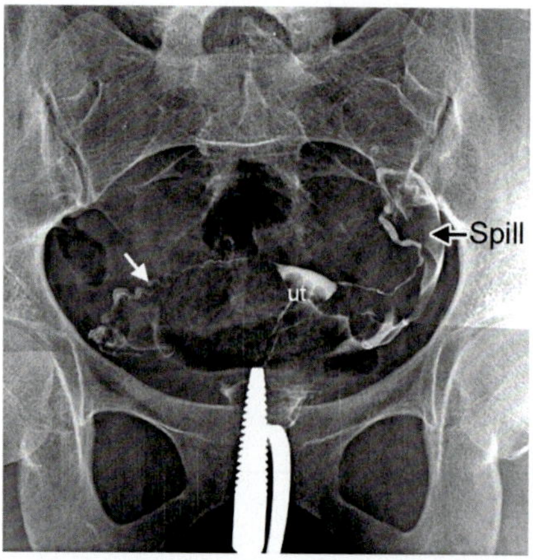


Fig. 8.1: Normal HSG shows normal uterus filled with contrast. Both fallopian tubes are filled with free peritoneal spill of contrast on both sides delineating the bowel loops

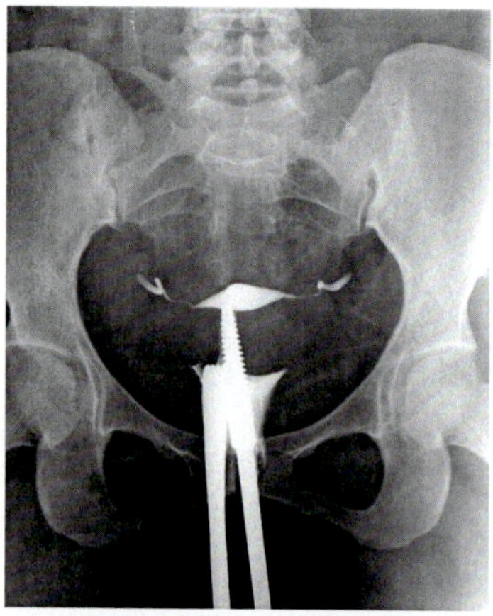

Fig. 8.2: HSG shows bilateral tubal block

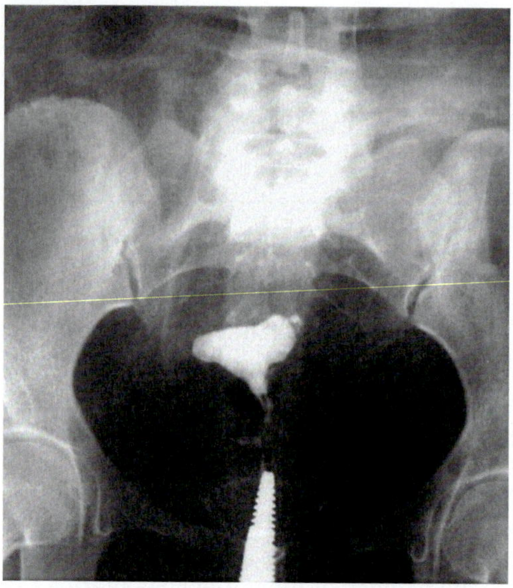

Fig. 8.3: HSG shows bilateral cornual occlusion

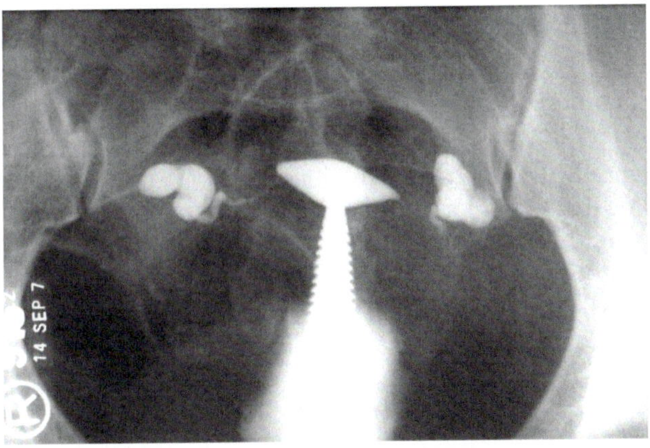


Fig. 8.4: HSG shows bilateral hydrosalpinx

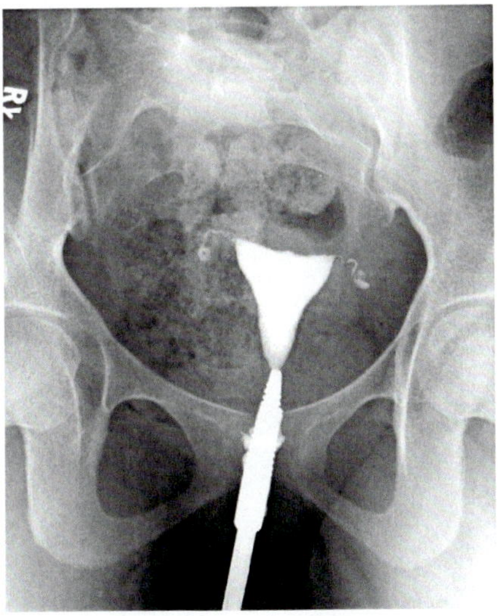

Fig 8.5: HSG shows bilateral tubectomy clips blocking the fallopian tubes, HSG performed for evaluation for tuboplasty

The purpose of the HSG is not therapeutic, but sometimes forcing the contrast through the tube may dislodge any material which blocks it, pregnany has taken place sometimes following a hysterosalpingogram without further treatment.

## UTERINE MALFORMATIONS

Abnormal development of the Mullerian ducts, during embryogenesis result in uterine malformation. Symptoms may be amenorrhea, infertility, pain and recurrent miscarriages depending on the nature of the defect. The incidence of uterine malformation is 6 to 7% in the general population. Uterine malformation may have associated renal abnormalities.

American Society of Reproductive Medicine has classified uterine malformation into six groups

1. Mullerian agenesis: Uterus is absent, vagina may be rudimentary or absent.
2. Unicornuate uterus is one-sided uterus where only one side of the Mullerian duct develops.
3. Uterus didelphys (uterus didelphis) is where both Mullerian ducts develop but fail to fuse, thus the patient has a double uterus (Figs 8.6A to C). This may be a condition with a double cervix and a vaginal partition, or the lower Mullerian system is fused and unpaired.

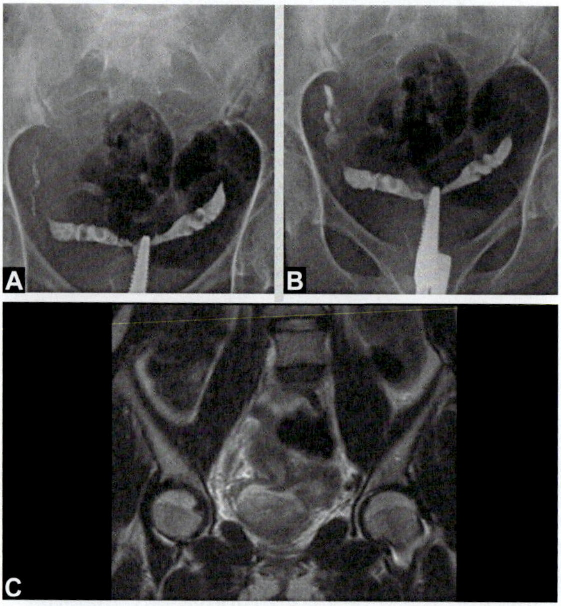

**Figs 8.6A to C:** (A and B) HSG shows uterus didelphys; (C) MRI of another patient shows uterus didelphys

4. Bicornuate uterus is uterus with two horns, in this only the upper part of that part of the Mullerian system that forms the uterus fails to fuse, the distal part of the uterus is normal, the proximal part is bifurcated giving it a heart-like appearance.
5. Septated uterus where the uterus is partitioned: In this, the two Mullerian ducts have fused, but the partition between them persists, splitting into two compartments.
6. DES (diethylstilbestrol) uterus is a "T-shape" uterine cavity as a result of fetal exposure to diethylstilbestrol.

An additional variation is the arcuate uterus where there is a concave dimple in the fundus of the uterus within the cavity.

## HYPOPLASTIC UTERUS

A 15-year-old girl referred because of primary amenorrhea was found to have a hypoplastic uterus measuring 36 x 10 x 13 mm (Figs 8.7A and B). The normal uterus is pear-shaped muscular organ located between the bladder and the rectum. The endometrial cavity is continuous with the cervical canal, and the two openings superiorly lead to the fallopian tubes. The average adolescent uterus is about 7.5 mm long, 5 mm wide and 2.5 mm thick. After menopause, the uterus shrinks to the pre-adolescent size.

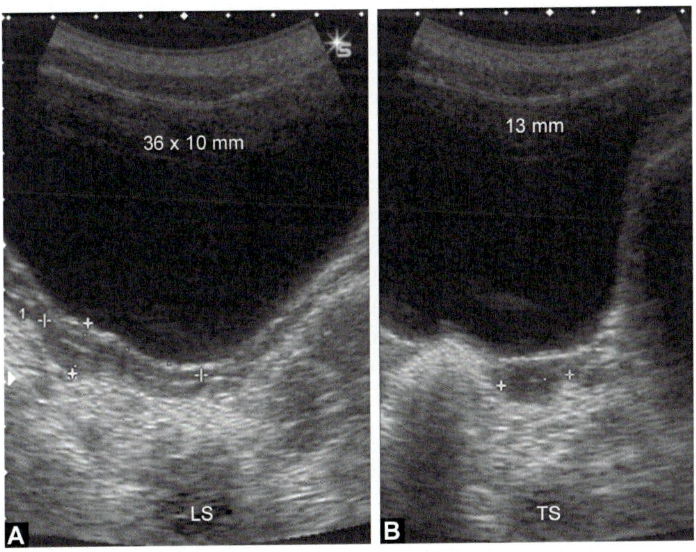


**Figs 8.7A and B:** (A) Ultrasound shows hypoplastic uterus which measures 36 × 10 mm in long section; (B) 13 mm thick in cross section

## ULTRASOUND IN FIRST TRIMESTER OF PREGNANCY

The benefits of the first trimester pregnancy scan include confirmation that the fetus is alive, accurate dating of the pregnancy, early diagnosis of major fetal defects, and the detection of multiple pregnancies and an important role in the assessment of increased nuchal translucency thickness and risk for trisomy 21. The early scan also provides reliable identification of chorionicity, which is the main determinant of outcome in multiple pregnancies.

### Scanning Technique

#### *Transabdominal Ultrasound*

The transabdominal ultrasound employs 3.5 MHz curvilinear probe and begins just above the pubic symphysis in a longitudinal axis. It is best performed when the patient has a full bladder, which not only provides a good window for viewing underlying structures, but also displaces overlying bowel.

#### *Transvaginal Ultrasound*

The transvaginal ultrasound is best performed on patients with an empty bladder to reduce patient discomfort and less uterine distortion from a distended bladder. The transvaginal probe is a 5 MHz probe and is covered with a probe condom.

### Ultrasound Findings

#### *Intrauterine Pregnancy*

The earliest sign of pregnancy seen with transvaginal ultrasound is the intradecidual sign, an anechoic sac without a distinct chorionic ring. This may be seen as early as four weeks of gestation. Definitive sonographic evidence of an intrauterine pregnancy is established when a gestational sac containing a yolk sac is identified in two planes within the endometrium. This occurs around the fifth week of gestation (Fig. 8.8).

In case of twin pregnancy (Fig. 8.9), if there are two separate placentas, the pregnancy is dichorionic, but, in the majority of cases, the two placentas are adjacent to each other and there are often difficulties in distinguishing between dichorionic-fused and monochorionic placentas.

In dichorionic twins, the intertwin membrane is composed of a central layer of chorionic tissue sandwiched between two layers of amnion, whereas in monochorionic twins there is no chorionic layer.

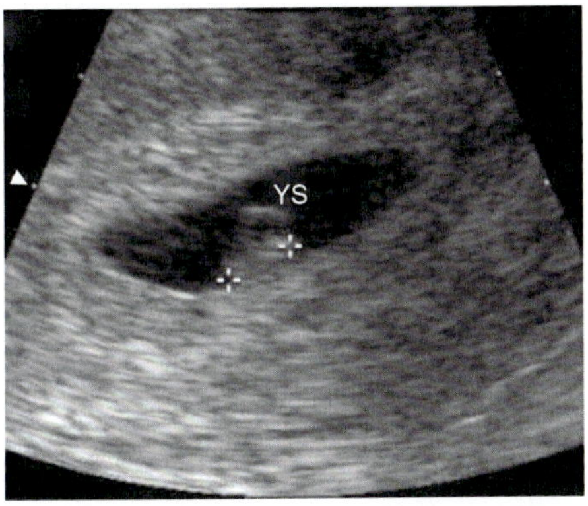


Fig. 8.8: Gestational sac is identified within the endometrium

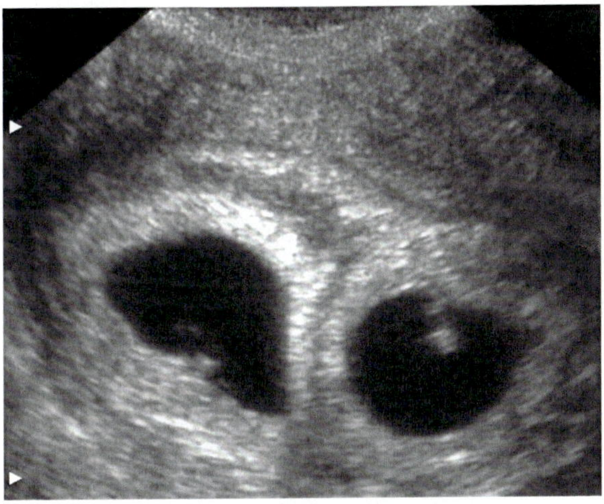

Fig. 8.9: Twin pregnancy

### Abnormal Pregnancy

Signs suggestive of abnormal embryonic development include a gestational sac greater than 10 mm in diameter without a visible yolk sac, a gestational sac greater than 18 mm in diameter without a fetal pole or a collapsed gestational sac. Additionally, when the difference between the mean sac diameter and crown rump length (CRL) is less than 5 mm, there is a significant risk of spontaneous abortion. Other signs associated with a poor prognosis include the absence of a fetal heart beat in an embryo with a CRL of at least 5 mm and a fetal heart beat less than 90 beats per minute. Gestational trophoblastic disease (molar pregnancy) may present with multiple, small, irregular cystic lesions within the endometrium.

### *Ectopic Pregnancy*

Ectopic pregnancy is the implantation of the blastocyst outside the endometrial lining of the uterus. This may occur within the peritoneal cavity, fallopian tubes, ovaries, and cervix or within a scar of prior uterine surgery. Ninety-five percent of all ectopic pregnancies occur within the fallopian tubes. The most definitive sonographic sign of ectopic pregnancy is the visualization of an extrauterine gestational sac containing a yolk sac, embryo or fetal heart beat. This occurs in approximately 14% of ectopic pregnancies.

## FOLLICULAR CYST

### Follicular Cysts

Follicular cysts are functional cysts, develop when a follicle fails to ovulate or involute. Majority of follicular cysts occurs in women of reproductive age-group. It is a simple unilocular cyst, round, anechoic structure with a thin wall casting posterior acoustic enhancement on ultrasound examination. The size of the cyst varies from 3 to 5 cm. Finding a follicular cysts is a common incidental finding seen as well-defined, rounded, unilocular, homogeneous, water density mass with smooth thin walls and low attenuation content (Fig. 8.10).

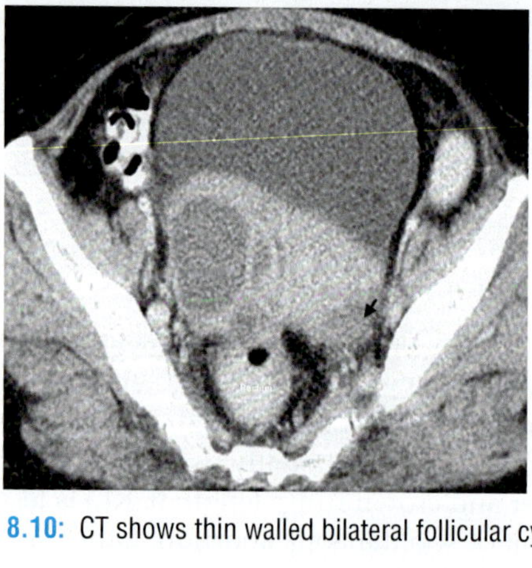

**Fig. 8.10:** CT shows thin walled bilateral follicular cysts

Simple follicular cysts usually resolve spontaneously. A follow-up ultrasound is recommended 6 weeks after initial imaging evaluation to see for cyst resolution.

The differential diagnosis of follicular cysts includes nonfunctional cysts and cystic neoplasm. Nonfunctional cysts include surface epithelial inclusion cysts, rete cysts and paraovarian and paratubal cysts.

## CORPUS LUTEUM CYST

Corpus luteal cysts are *functional cysts*, formed as a result of luteinization, after ovulation by the dominant follicle whose wall becomes vascularized, thickened and partially collapsed. They can result in periovulatory abdominal pain and may require imaging evaluation. Corpus luteal cysts are larger and symptomatic but less common than follicular cysts. Corpus luteal cysts are usually unilateral and more prone to hemorrhage and rupture. If the ovum is fertilized, the corpus luteum continues as the corpus luteum of pregnancy. It reaches its maximum size at 8 to 10 weeks and usually resolves spontaneously by 12 to 16 weeks. On ultrasound, it has a thick hyperechoic and finely scalloped wall. The contents are hyperechoic because of bleeding into the follicle that has ovulated and the wall has higher fat content resulting in hyperechoic wall. On Doppler, it shows a ring of fire appearance. Corpus luteal cyst on CT are thick walled unilocular cysts, measuring less than 3 cm in diameter with finely scalloped, hyperdense enhancing wall.

## FIBROID UTERUS

Fibroid (leiomyoma) uterus is a benign tumor that originates from the smooth muscle layer (myometrium) and the accompanying connective tissue of the uterus and can grow to a very large size. The location of leiomyoma may be submucosal, intramural, subserosal or cervical. It may be single or multiple. It may undergo hyaline, cystic or hemorrhagic degeneration and may show calcification. It occurs in 20% of premenopausal women. In fibroids malignant degeneration is rare. Symptoms are because of its location and its size as mass effect which include bleeding, heavy painful periods, abdominal discomfort, backache, urinary frequency, and infertility.

Ideal evaluation of uterine fibroid is magnetic resonance imaging (MRI) and ultrasound. Ultrasound is less expensive easy availability however MRI is superior and delineates the number, size and position of fibroids [Figs 8.11 and 8.12(A and B)]. Fibroids contain more collagen than normal uterine muscle and, as a result, the fibroids appear distinct and darker on the MRI. Leiomyomas are sharply marginated and are low signal intensity on T1 and T2 weighted images (Figs 8.13A and B). Degenerative fibroids give varied signal. The lesion is surrounded by pseudocapsule formed by neighboring tissue. The sensitivity of detecting fibroid on MRI is about 90%. MRI indicates and guides if a laparoscopic myomectomy is being considered.

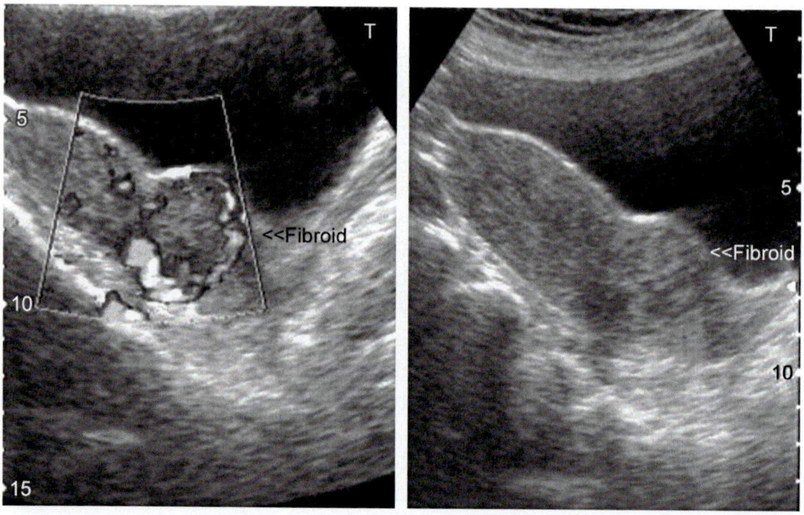


**Fig. 8.11:** Well defined hypoechoic mass in the lower part, anterior wall of uterus with central necrosis in a case of uterine fibroid

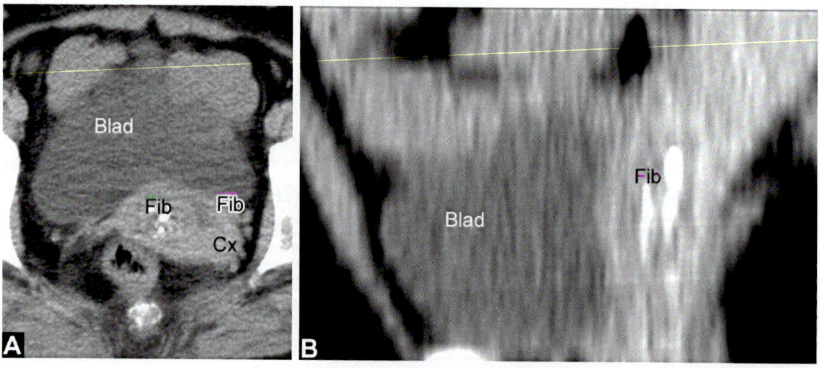


**Figs 8.12A and B:** Contrast enhanced CT pelvis images show a cervix mass with internal calcification in the region of cervix was confirmed as cervical fibroid

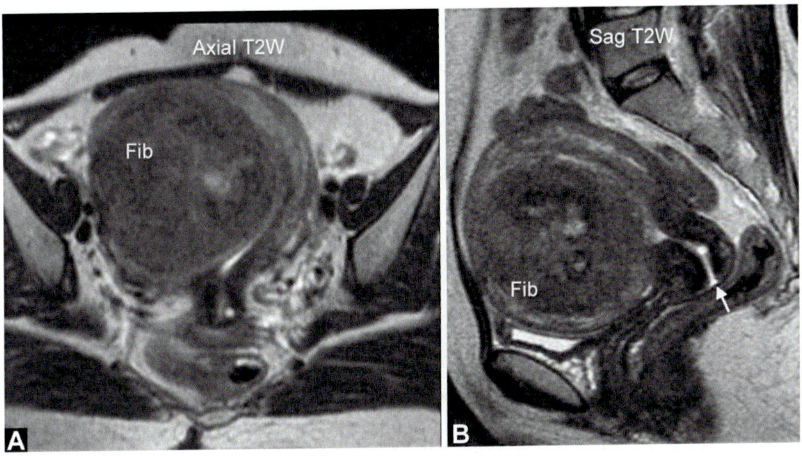


**Figs 8.13A and B:** MRI shows a large sharply marginated and low signal intensity mass on T1 and T2 weighted images involving fundus and body of uterus

## BROAD LIGAMENT FIBROID

Extrauterine fibroids though do occur, but are rare. Among the extrauterine fibroids, broad ligament fibroids are the most common. Because of its rarity it poses specific diagnostic difficulties (Figs 8.14A to D).

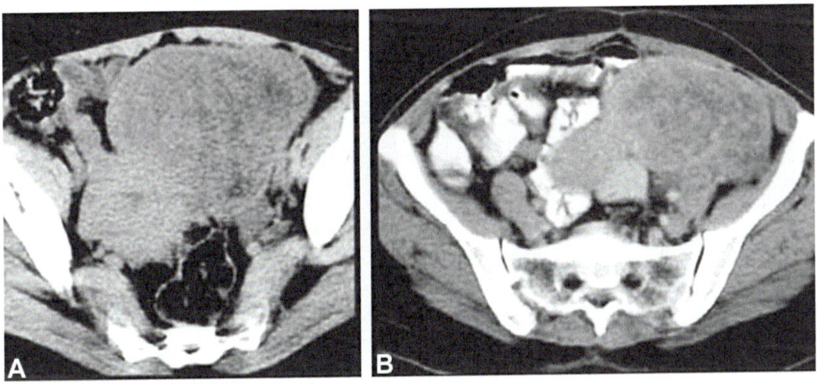


*Contd...*

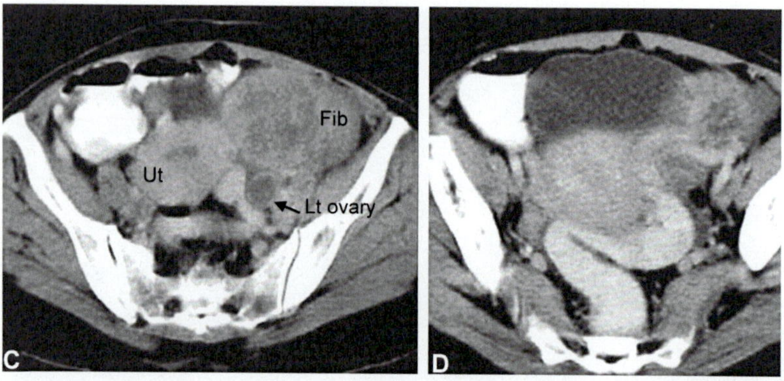


**Figs 8.14A to D:** CT Images show a moderately enhancing soft tissue density mass in left adnexa attached to superior lateral aspect of uterus. Left ovary is seen separately from the mass. This turned out to be a broad ligament fibroid on surgery

## PYOMETRA

Pyometra occurs when the natural drainage of the uterine cavity is compromised and pus accumulates within the cavity (Figs 8.15A and B). It is seen most frequently in postmenopausal women, but it can occur in younger women. Presenting symptoms include fever, vaginal discharge, postmenopausal bleeding, abdominal pain, and enlarged uterus. It seen associated with or is thought to signal the presence of an underlying malignancy of the genital tract. It may result from post irradiation resulting from radiation therapy for cervical cancer.

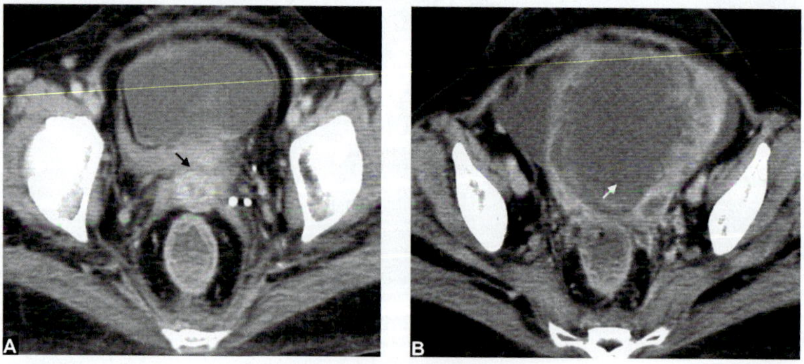


**Figs 8.15A and B:** Axial CT sections of pelvis do not show any obvious pelvic mass: (A) However, the cervical canal is stenosed (arrow); (B) Fluid collection is seen in the uterus (arrow). This was due to stenosis of cervix following radiotherapy for carcinoma of cervix

## OVARIAN CYST

The functional or retention cysts are due to failure of involution of follicle/corpus luteum with changes of menstrual cycle. The follicular cyst is the graffian follicle which fails to ovulate. The corpus luteum cyst is formed in postovulatory phase. These cysts regress spontaneously.

The imaging classification of ovarian cyst includes three types, simple cyst, hemorrhagic cyst and the complex cyst.

A *simple cyst* is seen on ultrasound as a unilocular thin walled less than 3 cm in diameter with anechoic contents and posterior acoustic enhancement. The color Doppler flow in cyst wall has pulsatility index more than 1.0 and resistive index (RI) more than 0.4. On MR imaging it appears isointense to urine in all sequences.

On ultrasound, the *hemorrhagic cyst* is seen as an echogenic mass, whirled pattern of mixed echogenicity or like fishnet. No color Doppler signal is seen within the cyst. On MR imaging, it shows intermediate to high signal on both T1 and T2 weighed images with distinct central hypointensity on T2 weighed images.

Any cyst which does not satisfy criteria for simple cyst or hemorrhagic cyst is called as a *complex cyst*. It may have internal septations, internal echoes or mural nodule showing color flow on Doppler study.

### Approach to ovarian cyst

#### A. Premenopausal woman

| Imaging finding | Management |
|---|---|
| Simple cyst < 2.5 cm | No follow up required |
| Simple cyst 2.5-6.0 cm | Clinical and ultrasound follow up in 2 months |
| Hemorrhagic cyst 2.5-6.0 cm | Clinical and ultrasound follow up in 1 month and hormonal treatment |
| Unilocular cyst > 6 cm | Surgery |

#### B. Postmenopausal woman

| Imaging finding | Management |
|---|---|
| Simple cyst | Serial follow up |
| Complex cyst, cyst > 3 cm, cyst with low RI (< 0.4) | CA 125 levels and surgical exploration |

## CARCINOMA OVARY

Carcinoma of the ovary is the second most common gynecological malignancy. They may be bilateral (Figs 8.16A and B). This is classified according to tissue of origin. Majority are epithelial tumors. Others include germ cell tumors, stromal-sex cord tumors and metastatic cancers from extraovarian primary sites. Incidence of these types varies widely. As per ten years data at one institute, epithelial tumors constitute 83 percent. According to another study epithelial ovarian carcinoma (Figs 8.17A and B) account for 90% of all ovarian malignancies. These are separated into two major categories; invasive (80%) and noninvasive or borderline (20%) tumors. Epithelial invasive cancers are further classified into serous cystadenocarcinoma (Figs 8.18A to D), mucinous cystadenocarcinoma, clear cell carcinoma and undifferentiated tumor. Ovarian carcinoma predominantly occurs in postmenopausal women and up to 85 percent of them present with peritoneal spread (Stage III).

Patients usually present with abdominal pain, distention or symptoms related to gastrointestinal tract or and genitourinary tract compression or nonspecific constitutional symptoms. A pelvic mass may be evident on abdominal palpation or pelvic examination but it is usually detected or confirmed on initial sonographic examination.

Spread of the tumor is transcoelomic and follows the pathways of peritoneal fluid circulation. Accordingly, deposits in right subdiaphrag-

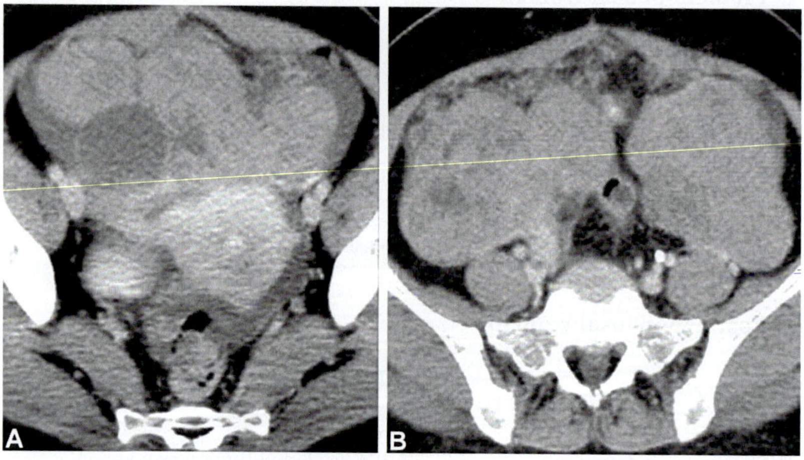


**Figs 8.16A and B:** (A) CT pelvis shows a uterus and adnexal masses; (B) Adnexal masses show mild enhancement

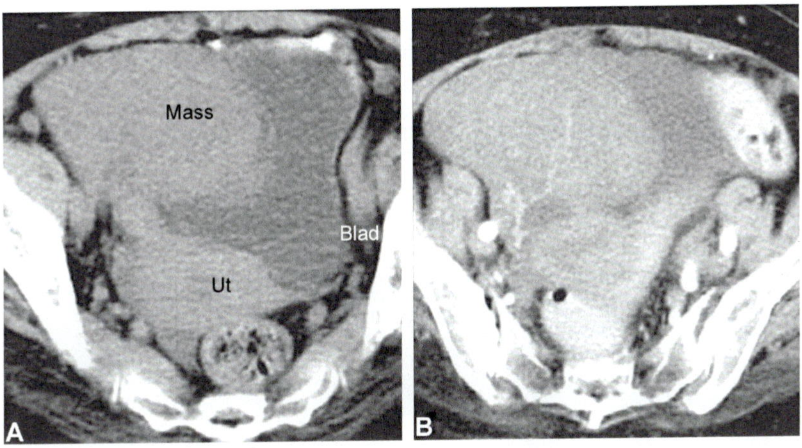


**Figs 8.17A and B:** Plain (A) and postcontrast (B) CT images show a feeding vessel (arrow) entering the right ovarian mass which turned out to be an undifferentiated epithelial ovarian malignancy

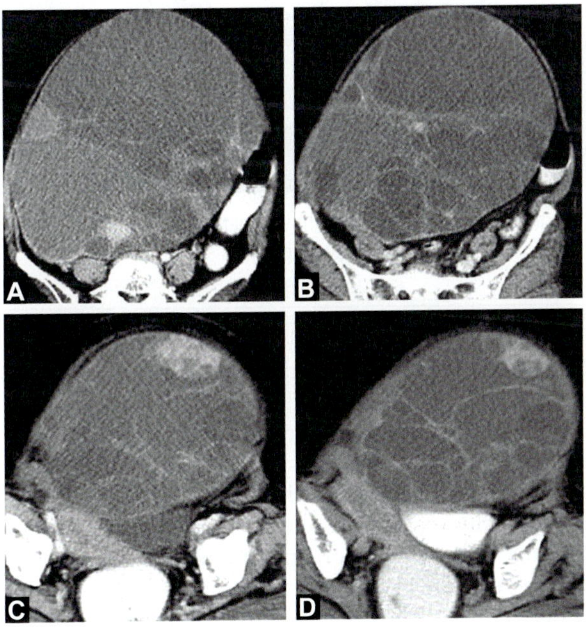


**Figs 8.18A to D:** Contrast CT shows a large cystic lesion with enhancing thick septae and enhancing mural nodules arising from right ovary confirmed as serous cystadenocarcinoma

matic region and para-colic gutters occur early along with ascites. Eventfully all peritoneal surfaces, omentum and mesentery may be involved. Metastases to the para-aortic and pelvis lymph nodes also occur.

## OVARIAN VEIN THROMBOSIS

Postpartum ovarian vein thrombosis (Fig. 8.19) is an uncommon complication of the postpartum period. CT angiography is the investigation of choice.

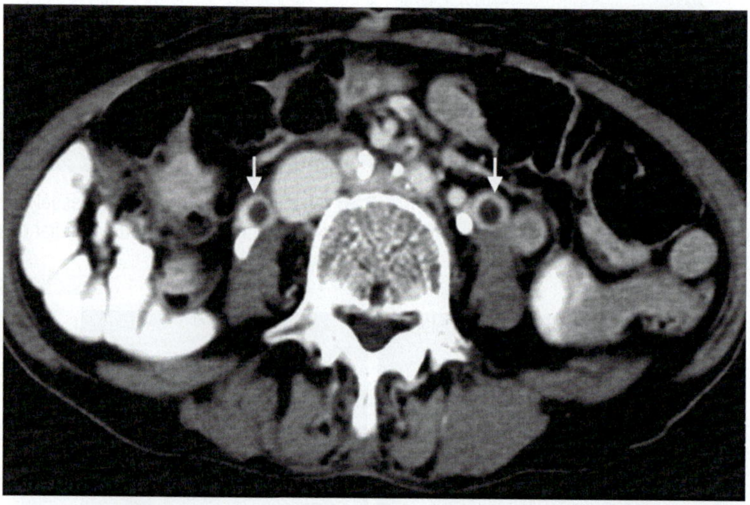

**Fig. 8.19:** Contrast-enhanced CT scan shows bilateral intravascular filling defect in the ovarian veins

## CARCINOMA OF ENDOMETRIUM

Prolonged estrogen stimulation is the main risk factor for endometrial cancer. An increased incidence of endometrial carcinoma is seen in women taking estrogen such as for oral contraception or postmenopausal women taking tamoxifen as a part of hormonal therapy for breast cancer. Other risk factors include nulliparity, obesity, and diabetes. The peak incidence of endometrial carcinoma is between the ages of 55 and 65 years.

Most patients present with postmenopausal vaginal bleeding or discharge, however, it can also occur in premenopausal women. In less than 5 percent of patients, the tumor is detected incidentally on cervical cytology or histopathology of uterus removed for benign causes. The diagnosis of endometrial carcinoma (Figs 8.20A to D) in suspected patients is made by histopathological examination of endometrial biopsy and curettage. Up to 90 percent of the endometrial cancers are adenocarcinoma, the rest include adenosquamous carcinoma, clear cell carcinoma and papillary serous carcinoma.

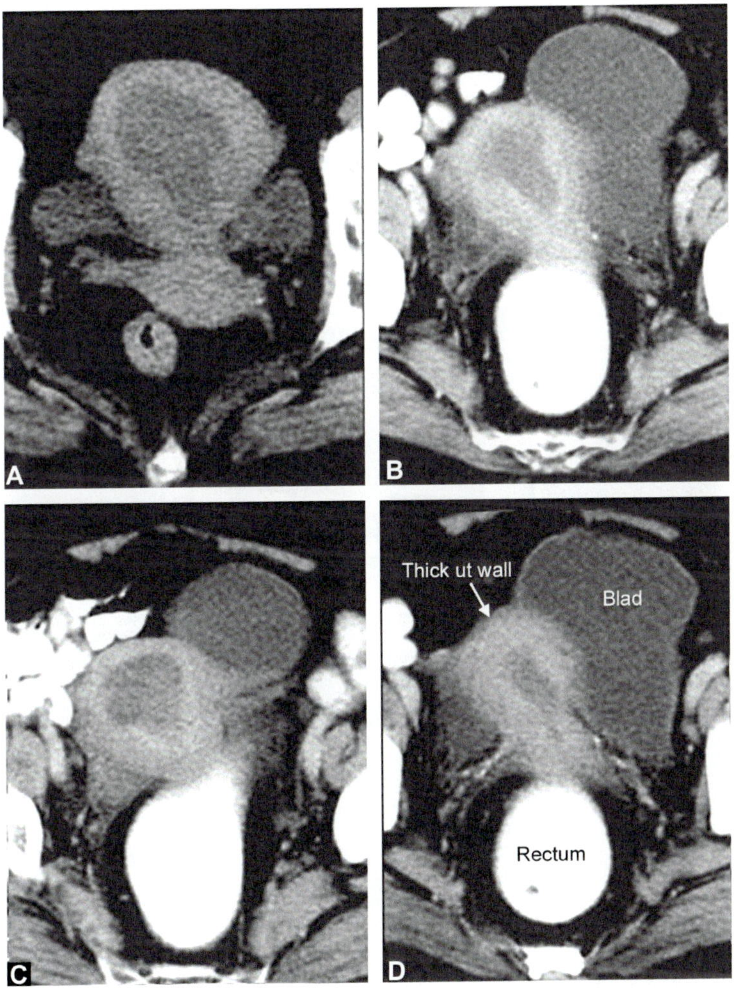


**Figs 8.20A to D:** CT pelvis shows collection in the uterine cavity lined on all sides by a thick irregular endometrial wall. Biopsy proved this to be a high grade endometrial carcinoma

## CARCINOMA CERVIX

In cervical carcinoma, the cervix becomes enlarged and irregular, it enhances less than the surrounding normal cervical tissue. If the cervical canal is obstructed there may be fluid in the uterine cavity which will be distended.

Carcinoma cervix is better demonstrated on MRI than on X-ray, ultrasound and CT (Figs 8.21 to 8.23). CT has limited role in staging due to poor tissue discrimination and difficulty in discriminating adjacent organ involvement whereas MRI has over 90% accurateness in staging. Parametrial invasion is displayed by an eccentric soft-tissue mass and stranding into the surrounding fat. Loss of the fat planes between the cervix with the rectum or bladder or ureters indicate stage 3. The treatment and prognosis of cervical carcinoma depends on volume, extent, vascular, lymphatic spread and histology.

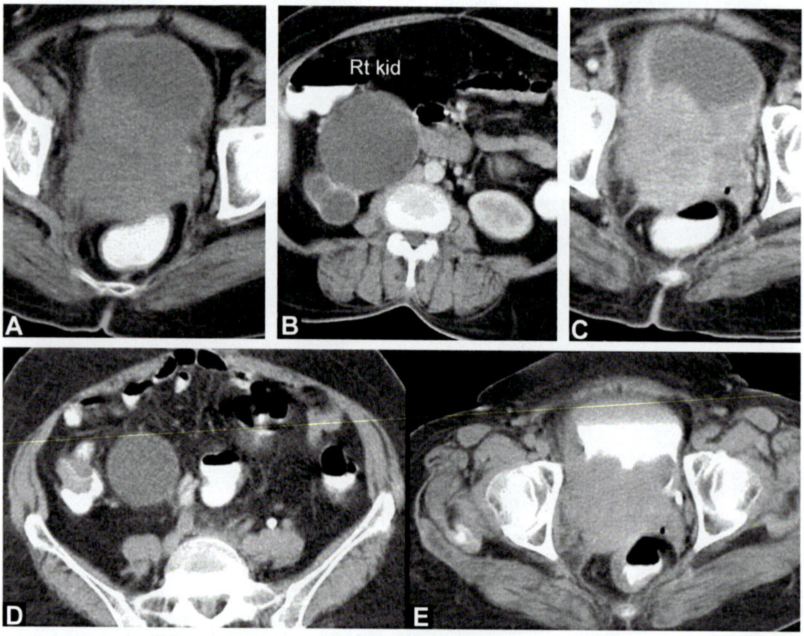


**Figs 8.21A to E:** (A) Plain CT abdomen-pelvis shows a hyperdense cervical mass with loss of fat plane anteriorly with urinary bladder and posteriorly with rectum; (B) Immediate postcontrast CT shows normal contrast uptake by left kidney. Right kidney shows gross hydronephrosis; (C to E) show invasion of the uterus, urinary bladder, rectum and right lower ureter

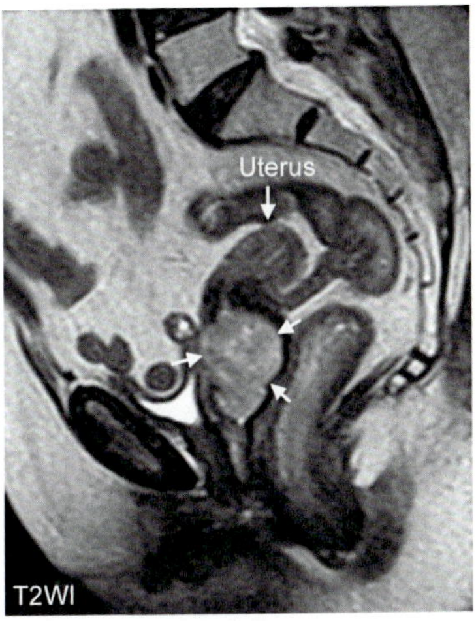


Fig. 8.22: Carcinoma cervix on MRI present as a soft tissue mass lesion in the cervix (arrows), It appears hyperintense on T2W image

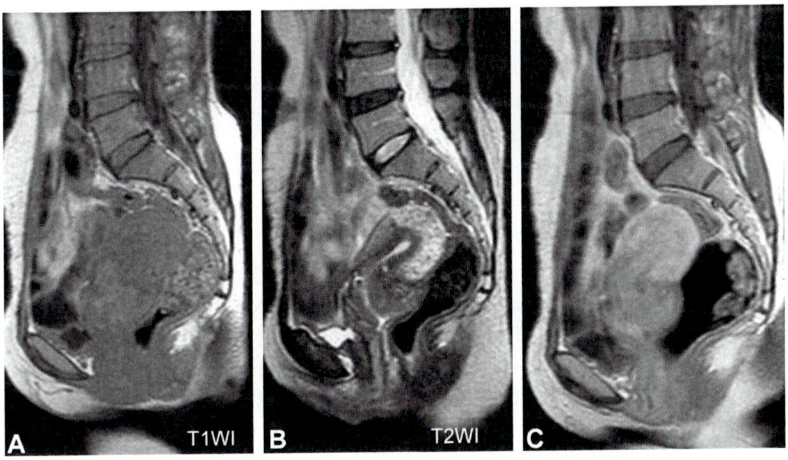


Figs 8.23A to C: Carcinoma cervix in a 40 years old female who presented with history of PV bleeding of 12 days duration. Cervix is bulky and reveals altered heterogeneous signal. It is iso-to-mildly hyperintense on T1W image (A) and iso-to-hypointense on T2W image (B). It shows heterogeneous enhancement (C). The posterior wall is predominantly involved. The lower uterine segment is also involved. The fibrous stroma appears to be intact. Biopsy confirmed as adenocarcinoma

## IMAGING IN ASSISTED REPRODUCTION

Infertility refers to the state of a woman who is unable to carry a pregnancy to full term. Infertility may also as per WHO guidelines consider a couple infertile and eligible for treatment if a woman under 35 has not conceived after 12 months of contraceptive-free intercourse or a woman over 35 has not conceived after 6 months of contraceptive-free sexual intercourse.

Primary infertility means that couple has never been able to conceive and secondary infertility is difficulty in conceiving after already having conceived.

Specific female infertility causes are:

- Ovulation problems
- Tubal blockage
- Age-related factors
- Uterine problems
- Previous tubal ligation.

Imaging techniques regularly employed in assisted reproduction:

1. Gray scale ultrasonography
2. Doppler ultrasound
3. Sonohysterography
4. Hysterosalpingography.

### Monitoring Treatment

#### *Confirming Downregulation*

The first stage of many Assisted Reproductive Technologies (ART) cycles, prior to ovarian stimulation, is to obtain control over the hypothalamic–pituitary–ovarian axis through the induction of pituitary downregulation. Downregulation is assessed ultrasonographically by demonstrating relatively inactive ovaries with no large follicles ($\geq$10 mm) in association with a thin endometrium ($\leq$5 mm) and a low estradiol level. The 3D ultrasound allows the endometrial volume to be measured accurately, but the evidence so far has failed to show that this offers any additional benefits.

### Follicular Development

Once downregulation has been achieved, exogenous gonadotropin is administered subcutaneously. Supraphysiological doses are given in an attempt to recruit multiple follicles from the selectable antral follicle population and to support their continued development into preovulatory follicles that contain mature oocytes capable of being fertilized. Mature oocytes are generally recovered from follicles with a mean diameter of ≥14 mm, but may be obtained from smaller follicles. As fertilization rates are also lower with oocytes derived from large follicles (≥24 mm), a compromise has to be made. Most units aim to undertake oocyte collection when there are at least three follicles measuring ≥17–18 mm, although the criteria of individual units vary considerably.

Ultrasonography is regarded as a safe, accurate and efficient method of monitoring follicular development in response to ovarian stimulation and is an essential part of the process. Recent developments have seen the introduction of automated measurement of follicles, which has implications for standardization and work flow. Sono-AVC (Automatic Volume Calculation) identifies and quantifies hypoechoic regions within a 3D data set and provides automatic estimation of their absolute dimensions, mean diameter and volume. As each different volume is separately color-coded, Sono-AVC is an ideal tool for the study of follicular development within the ovary.

### Ultrasound-guided Procedures

Ultrasound is used to direct the transvaginal collection of oocytes and the subsequent transfer of embryos into the uterus. Once correct positioning of the needle tip in the center of each follicle has been confirmed, gentle suction is applied and the follicular fluid is aspirated into a test tube through a closed system. Follicular flushing has been traditionally employed in the belief that it may improve the oocyte yield, although this may not improve the number of oocytes retrieved and increases the duration of retrieval and postoperative pain. If the first aspirate does not contain an oocyte, the follicle is flushed several times until one is seen in the aspirate or the observer moves on to the next follicle. The procedure is repeated until all of the large follicles have been aspirated.

Embryo transfer generally takes place two to three days after oocyte recovery, but may be delayed for five days in the case of blastocyst transfer. One or two embryos are placed into the uterus by passing a fine, flexible catheter through the cervix into the endometrial cavity. Ultrasound may be used to guide the embryo transfer and the evidence suggests that this improves success rates if the embryos are deposited 1 to 2 cm below the uterine fundus.

# 9

# CHAPTER

# Central Nervous System

**Chapter Outline**

- Extradural Hematoma
- Meningomyelocele
- Neurogenic Tumors
- Cold Abscess
- Thyroglossal Cyst
- Dental and Dentigerous Cyst

## EXTRADURAL HEMATOMA

Extradural hematoma is collection of blood in the extradural space which lies between the dura and skull vault. It is also known as epidural hematoma. Usually, it is associated with fracture of temporoparietal region and is due to injury to middle meningeal artery or vein. It can be unilateral or bilateral.

### Clinical Features

There is history of transient loss of consciousness following a blow or fall. External injury and swelling may be seen in the temporal region of scalp. Patient soon regains consciousness and yet again after 6 to 12 hours (lucid interval) starts deteriorating. Later, the patient presents with confusion, irritability, drowsiness, hemiparesis on same side of the injury. Initially there is papillary constriction and later papillary dilatation occurs on the same side, finally the patient becomes unconscious.

X-ray skull may show fracture of temporal bone. CT brain is diagnostic. Extradural hematoma appears as a biconvex lesion which appears hyperdense, i.e. bright in the acute stage (Figs 9.1A and B) or hypodense, i.e. dark in the chronic stage. Associated contusions, intraparenchymal hematoma, fracture of bony calvarium and scalp swelling can also be appreciated.

Treatment is craniotomy to evacuate hematoma. Antibiotics and anticonvulsants are given postoperatively.

### Complications

a. Post-traumatic epilepsy
b. Meningitis
c. Post-traumatic amnesia.

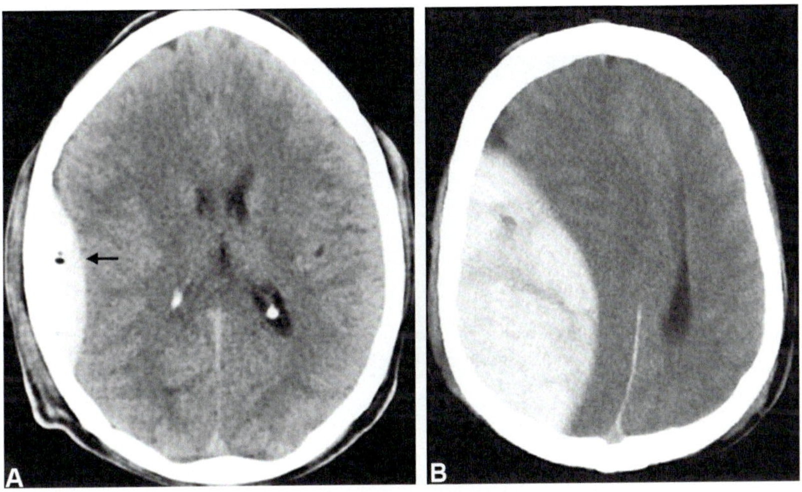


**Figs 9.1A and B:** (A) Plain CT brain shows right biconvex extradural hematoma with small loculated air inside (arrow); (B) In another case CT brain shows a massive left biconvex extradural hematoma

## MENINGOMYELOCELE

Meningomyelocele is the most common type of spinal dysraphism with incidence of two per thousand live births. In meningomyelocele superficial ectoderm does not separate from the neuroectoderm thereby producing a midline defect, the neural tube remains open and the neural folds remain in continuity with the cutaneous ectoderm at the skin surface. There is a sac covered by leptomeninges containing CSF and variable amount of neural tissue herniated through a defect in the posterior/anterior elements of spine. Most common location is thoracolumbar junction.

X-ray reveals the bony defect in the neural arch in the form of absent spinous process or widening of interpedicular distance. USG is primarily useful in the antenatal diagnosis and can detect open widened neural arch with flared laminae. It can show meningomyelocele sac and detect hydrocephalus and other associated cranial anomalies. Direct sonography of the sac using high frequency transducer in infants can provide similar information.

MRI detects cord abnormalities in addition to the detail evaluation of the content of the sac (Figs 9.2A and B). Repair of the defect can be done within 48 hours.

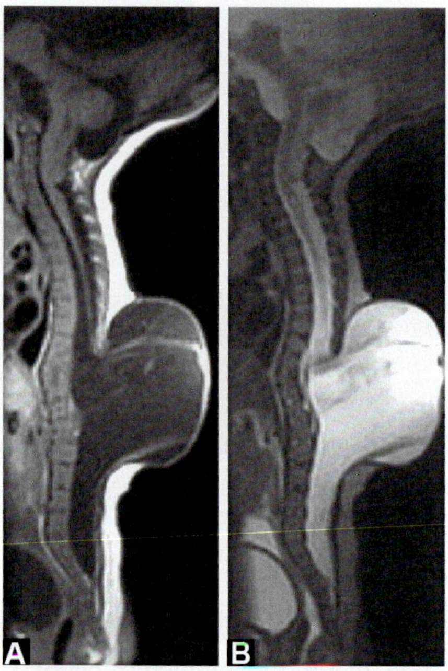


**Figs 9.2A and B:** Dorsolumbar meningomyelocele in a one-day-old male (body) presented with swelling on the back, MRI on sagittal T1W (A) T2W (B) Axial images show midline defect in the posterior elements of D9 to L2 vertebrae. A CSF filled sac is seen protruding through this defect beyond the plane of the back. It is not covered with skin. The spinal cord continues into the sac and the neural placode is adherent to the posterior aspect of the sac. Nerve roots are seen traversing through it

## NEUROGENIC TUMORS

Neurogenic tumors account for 16% of mediastinal tumors; about 10% of neurogenic tumors invade the spinal canal, and are called dumbbell tumors because of their shape. Surgery is the first-choice of treatment, in these cases surgical resection is difficult because it expands outside and inside the spinal canal via the intervertebral foramen.

Neurofibroma arises from nonspecific cells in the nerve sheath. It is a benign expansile lesion through which the nerve passes (Figs 9.3A and B). When it grows in size it enlarges the foramina through which it passes (dumb-bell tumor) or contiguous bones undergo pressure erosion leading to bony defect. On MRI, neurofibromas have intermediate signal intensity on T1-weighted images, very high signal intensity on T2-weighted images and following gadolinium enhancement (Figs 9.4A to D).

Neuroblastomas can arise from anywhere along the sympathetic chain from primitive neural crest cells that differentiate to form the sympathetic nervous system and consist predominantly of neuroblasts, whereas ganglioneuromas are composed entirely of well-differentiated cells.

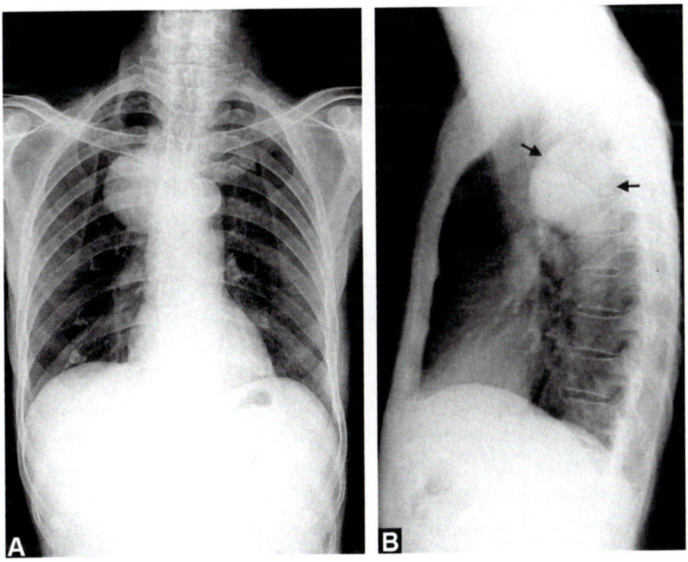

**Figs 9.3A and B:** X-ray Chest PA and lateral views show a well defined rounded posterior mediastinal mass overlying the thoracic vertebrae, suggestive of a neurogenic tumor (arrow)

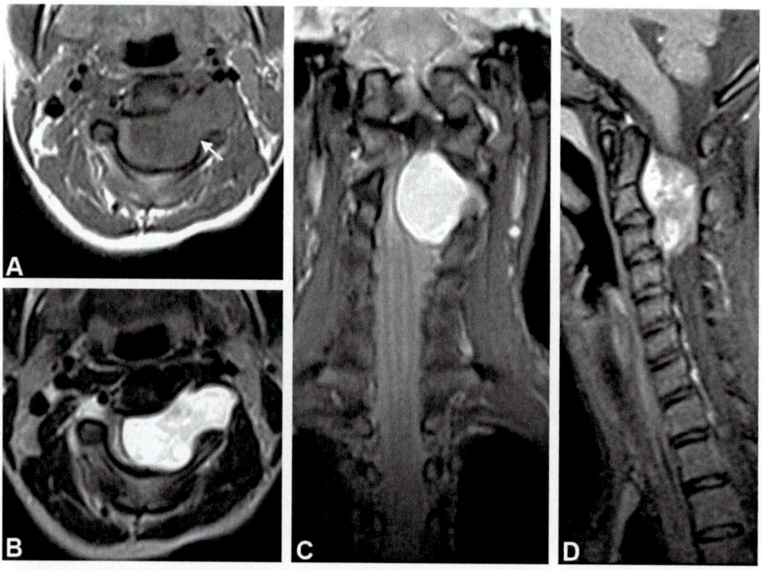

**Figs 9.4A to D:** A well defined dumb-bell shaped lesion is seen in the spinal canal, left neural foramen and left paraspinal region. The left neural foramen is widened. It is hypointense on T1: (A) Hyperintense on T2; (B) Shows moderate homogeneous enhancement on postcontrast T1W images; (C) Coronal T2W; (D) Image reveals compression and displacement of the cord to right

## COLD ABSCESS

A cold abscess is an abscess that commonly occurs due to tuberculosis. It develops so slowly that there is little inflammation, and it becomes painful only when there is pressure on the adjacent organs. It is most commonly located in the spine, hips, lymph nodes, or in the genital region but can occur anywhere.

Plain X-rays may show erosion of bone adjacent to the abscess, or may present as mass effect on adjacent organs, soft tissue swelling, displacement and blurring of fat planes. Newer imaging techniques are more helpful as compared to conventional X-rays.

Cold abscess may present with a sinus, sinogram will demonstrate the extent of the abscess. Ultrasonography helps to localize and show extent of the abscess. CT scan is more accurate showing extent of the abscess and bony changes if any.

Treatment is by drainage of the abscess by USG or CT-guided percutaneous catheter. Surgical drainage is recommended especially when percutaneous catheter drainage is not successful, followed by appropriate antibiotic therapy.

## Caries Spine

Caries spine or tubercular spine can occur at any age and present with spinal pain, local tenderness, limitation of spinal mobility and may develop paraplegia because of involvement of vertebrae and intervertebral disks, may develop paravertebral abscess or intraspinal extension of the lesion.

In caries spine, the intervertebral disk is frequently involved and there is frequent development of cold abscess which is seen on X-ray as displacement of psoas muscles or can be appreciated if calcification is present. Cold abscess is well appreciated on CT scan and MRI as a paravertebral lesion (Figs 9.5A to E). In caries spine, the intervertebral disk is most often involved with destruc-tion and resultant narrowing.

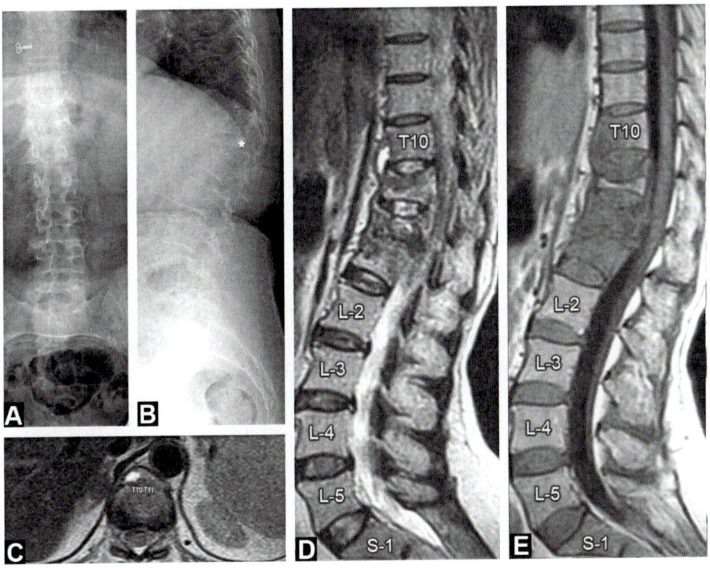


**Figs 9.5A to E:** (A and B) AP and lateral views of dorsolumber spine show wedge-shaped collapse of D11 vertebral body (*) with questionable paravertebral abscess; (C to E) MRI confirms the finding of X-ray and show destruction of D11 to L1 vertebral bodies and disks with anterior paravertebral abscess

X-ray spine may show the site of involvement, which may be:

1. Paradiskal: The disease most often begins in the vertebral body either superiorly or inferiorly adjacent to endplate.
2. Central: The disease process starts in the center of body which is seen as a lytic area with absence of trabeculae. This gradually enlarges and the vertebral body may expand and at a later stages result in concentric collapse.
3. Anterior subperiosteal: Infection begins at anterior vertebral margin underneath the periosteum and spreads beneath the anterior longitudinal ligament.
4. Appendiceal: The disease process involves neural arch that includes spinous process, laminae, transverse process and pedicle.

CT scan and MRI demonstrates bone destruction even when X-rays are normal. It shows bone destruction which may be fragmentary, osteolytic (Figs 9.5A to E), subperiosteal or sclerotic in nature.

## THYROGLOSSAL CYST

Thyroglossal cyst is a congenital cyst which presents as a swelling in the neck along the line of thyroglossal tract due to degeneration of a part of the tract. Most common location of thyroglossal cyst is subhyoid region. Other locations can be:

a. Foramen cecum
b. Floor of mouth
c. Suprahyoid
d. Thyroid cartilage.

Thyroid gland is usually present in the normal location or may be present in the wall of the thyroglossal cyst in that case the thyroid fossa is empty. Thyroglossal cyst presents as a swelling in the midline, which moves with deglutition. If infected it develops into an abscess. It may rarely under go a malignant change.

USG neck is diagnostic which reveals cystic nature of the lesion and rules out the differential diagnosis of a pretracheal lymph node or dermoid cyst. Radioisotope study shows absence or presence of thyroid tissue.

Treatment is by Sistrunk operation.

## DENTAL AND DENTIGEROUS CYST

Dental cyst is a unilocular cyst seen in relation to the chronically infected caries tooth and dentigerous cyst is unilocular cystic (Figs 9.6A and B) swelling arising in relation to the dental epithelium from an unerrupted tooth. It is seen at the crown of unerupted tooth usually premolars or molars.

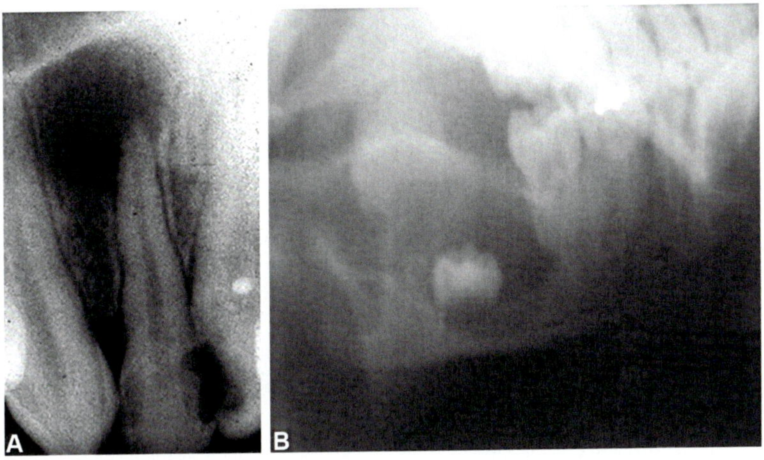

**Figs 9.6A and B:** (A) Dental cyst; (B) Dentigerous cyst

Difference between dental cyst and dentigerous cyst:

| Dental cyst | Dentigerous cyst |
|---|---|
| Also known as radicular or periapical cyst. It is the most common cyst of the jaw | Also known as follicular odontome |
| Unilocular cyst seen in relation to the chronically infected caries tooth | It is unilocular cystic swelling arising in relation to the dental epithelium from an unerrupted tooth. It is seen at the crown of unerrupted tooth usually premolars or molars |
| Clinical features-Presents as a tender swelling with expansion of the jaw | Clinical features-Painless, smooth and hard swelling in the jaw |
| Complication-Superadded infection leads to osteomyelitis of jaw | Complication—may undergo malignant transformation into ameloblastoma |
| Radiographic appearance<br>Round or pear-shaped unilocular periapical lucent lesion at the apex of nonvital tooth | Radiographic appearance<br>Well defined round or ovoid corticated lucent lesion with root of the lesion often outside the lesion |
| Treatment:<br>1. Antibiotics<br>2. Drainage or cyst excision | Treatment:<br>1. Excision of small cyst<br>2. Marsupialization for larger cyst |

# 10 CHAPTER

# Soft Tissues

**Chapter Outline**

- Costal Cartilage Calcification
- Dermoid Cysts
- Guinea Worm
- Sarcoidosis
- Seminal Vesicle Calcification
- Soft Tissue Calcification
- Breast Screening
- Carcinoma *In Situ*
- Lipoma

## COSTAL CARTILAGE CALCIFICATION

Costal cartilage calcification can help in distinguishing the sex. Calcification of costal cartilage may be seen above the age of 20 years in male and above the age of 16 years in females.

Pattern of calcification is peripheral (marginal) in males, it is mainly confined to the upper and lower margins of the costal cartilages (Figs 10.1A to D). In female, it is solid tongue-like protrusion of calcification, it is central pyramidal (lingular) type of calcification with beak towards sternum. Costocondral calcification is marginal in males and central in female.

## DERMOID CYSTS

Dermoid cysts (or mature cystic teratomas) are benign germ cell tumors composed of mature epithelial elements, i.e. skin, hair, desquamated epithelium, and teeth. They have wider age distribution, but most commonly occur in age group of 16 to 55 years. Malignant dermoid cysts are rare and usually develop into squamous cell carcinoma in adults; in children it usually develops into endodermal sinus tumor.

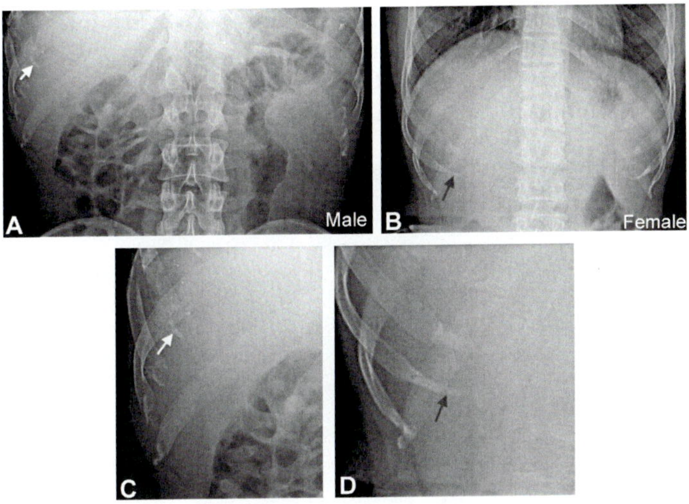


Figs 10.1A to D: X-rays of lower chest show costal cartilage calcification pattern of the lower ribs is that of a male and female

*Types of dermoid cysts are:*

1. Sequestration dermoids are caused when skin and skin structures become trapped during fetal development at the line of embryonic fusion. Common sites are forehead, head (Fig. 10.2), root of nose and sublingual dermoid.

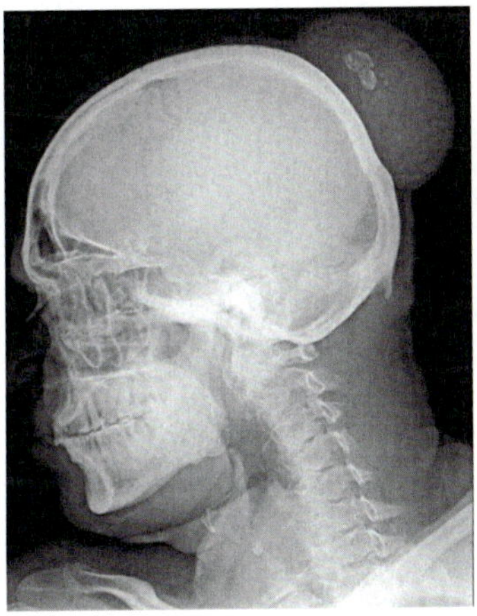

Fig. 10.2: X-ray of skull shows calcification in a sequestration dermoid in the scalp

2. Implantation dermoid occurs as epidermis gets buried into the deeper subcutaneous tissue due to minor pricks or trauma, which causes reaction and cyst formation. Common sites are fingers, toes and feet [Figs 10.3(A and B) and 10.4(A and B)].

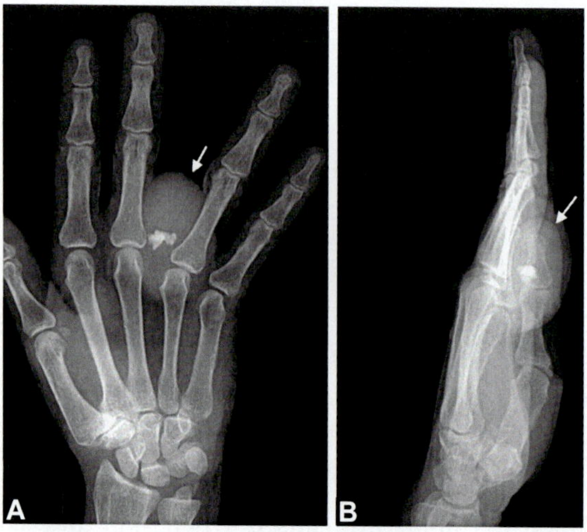


**Figs 10.3A and B:** X-rays of hand show implantation dermoid with calcification

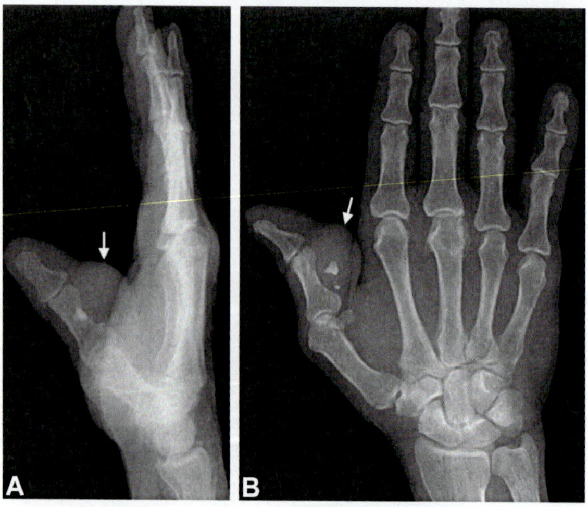


**Figs 10.4A and B:** X-rays of hand show calcification within the implantation dermoid over proximal phalanx of the thumb

3. Teratomatous dermoid occurs in ovary, testis, retroperitoneum and mediastinum.

Ultrasound (US) is the initial imaging investigation of choice. On US, it is smooth-walled cystic structure with varying internal composition depending upon mixture of epithelial elements. On CT, well defined cystic appearance with fat content and calcification (e.g. tooth) is suggestive of a dermoid.

## GUINEA WORM

### Calcified Guinea Worm

Guinea worm disease (Dracunculiasis) has been eradicated from Asia. In India, the last reported case was in July 1996 and on completion of three years of zero incidences, India was declared free from guinea worm disease. In this case, infestation must have taken place before eradication. Transmission of dracunculiasis now occurs in only few African countries.

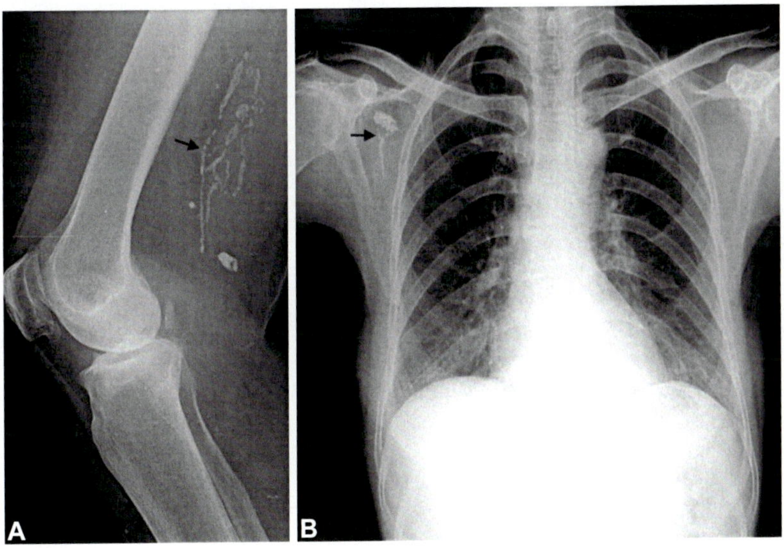


**Figs 10.5A and B:** (A) Knee X-ray shows string like calcified guinea worms in the soft tissues of the distal posterior aspect of thigh; (B) Chest X-ray shows calcified guinea worms as a high density string like calcification in the soft tissues of the right axilla in the same patient

Man acquires infection by drinking water containing infected cyclops. In the stomach, these cyclops are digested by gastric juice and the parasites are released. They penetrate the duodenal wall; migrate through viscera to the subcutaneous tissues of the various parts of the body. They grow into adults into 9 to 12 months. The female grows to a length of 55 to 120 cm, and the male is very short 2 to 3 cm. After infestation many of these parasites (usually gravid female, as male dies) emerge out through skin, while few of them are lodged in the subcutaneous tissues, die, get encapsulated and get calcified as string like appearance [Figs 10.5(A and B) and 10.6(A to D)]. Upon contact with water, the female parasite releases up to one million, microscopic larvae which remain active in water for 3 to 6 days. They are picked up by small crustaceans called cyclops. The larvae require a period of about 15 days for development in cyclops, which is the intermediate host.

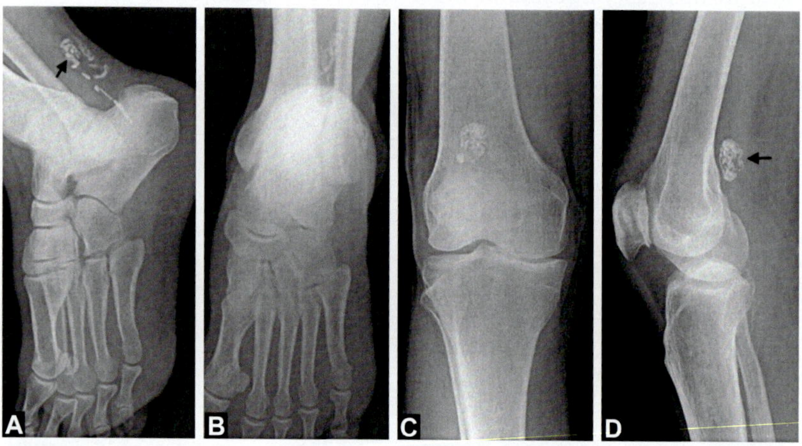


**Figs 10.6A to D:** X-rays ankle show: (A and B) Calcified guinea worms as a high density string like calcification in the soft tissues of the posterior aspect of ankle; (C and D) Posterior aspect of knee in another patient

## SARCOIDOSIS

Sarcoidosis commonly develops thoracic lymphadenopathy and parenchymal lung opacities. Adenopathy almost always precedes pulmonary shadowing, but they are often present simultaneously. The chest radiograph is abnormal at some time in 90% of patients with sarcoidosis. In sarcoidosis, there is bilateral symmetrical hilar enlargement involving both tracheobronchial and bronchopulmonary nodes. Bilateral hilar adenopathy in the correct clinical setting is considered as sufficient evidence of sarcoidosis and negate the need of biopsy, more so if they show presence of egg shell calcification (Fig. 10.7).

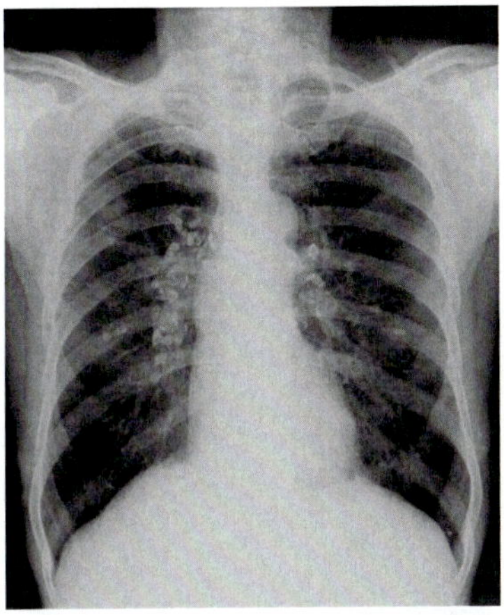

**Fig. 10.7:** X-ray chest shows multiple enlarged bilaterally symmetrical hilar lymph nodes which show peripheral or egg shell calcification

Enlargement of other mediastinal nodes are rarely appreciated on the chest radiograph but may be seen on CT. If the hilar adenopathy is very asymmetrical or anterior mediastinal adenopathy is present alternative diagnosis should be considered. The involved lymph nodes may undergo calcification, when this calcification is in the periphery it is referred as egg-shell calcification.

*Other causes of bilateral hilar lymphadenopathy:*

1. Infections like tuberculosis, mycoplasma, Whipple's disease.
2. Lymphoma, carcinoma, mediastinal tumors.
3. Organic dust diseases like silicosis, berylliosis.
4. Extrinsic allergic alveolitis like bird fancier's disease.
5. Less common causes like Churg-Strauss syndrome, human immunodeficiency virus, extrinsic allergic alveolitis, pneumoconiosis, adult onset Still's disease.

## SEMINAL VESICLE CALCIFICATION

The seminal vesicles are paired lobulated pouches, 5 cm in length (Fig. 10.8) but become atrophic with age. They lie on the posterior surface of urinary bladder. They run inferomedially into a thin duct and join with the duct of the vas deferens to form the ejaculatory duct. The ejaculatory duct penetrates the prostate to enter the prostatic urethra on the verumontanum.

Calcification of the seminal vesicles is uncommon phenomenon. Calcifications appear more frequently in diabetic patients (Fig. 10.9). Other causes of seminal vesicle calcification are recurrent urinary tract infection and paraplegia with chronic infection.

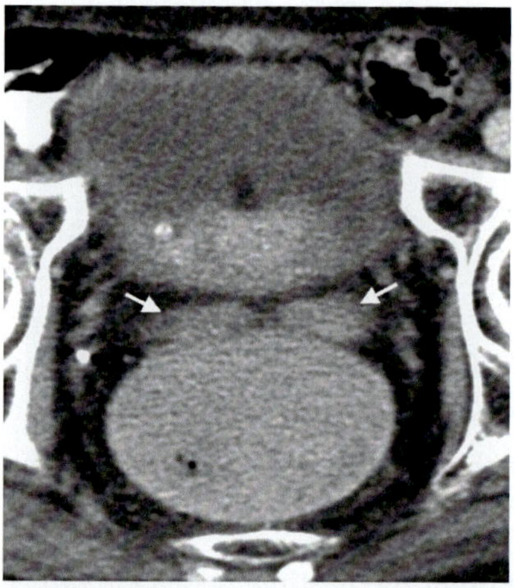

**Fig. 10.8:** CT of pelvis shows normal seminal vesicles as moustache-shaped structures

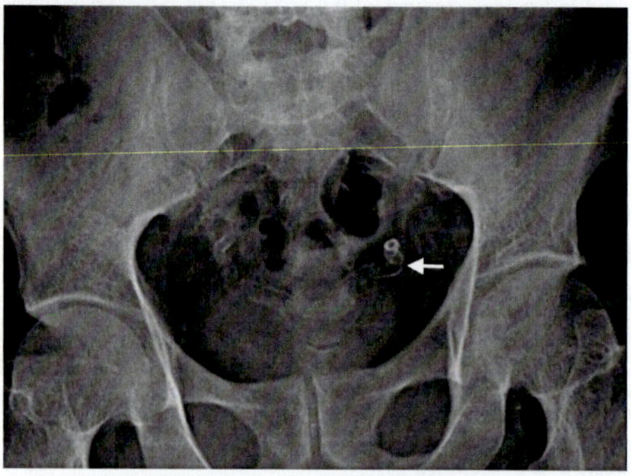

**Fig. 10.9:** X-ray of pelvis shows calcification of both seminal vesicles in a case of diabetes mellitus (arrow)

## SOFT TISSUE CALCIFICATION

Soft tissues calcification is frequently seen on conventional X-rays.

Soft tissue calcification is seen in pseudohypoparathyroidism (Fig. 10.10), thyroid adenomas, carcinoma thyroid (Figs 10.11A and B), tuberculous glands in the neck (Fig. 10.12), mediastinum or abdomen, neurofibromatosis (Figs 10.13A and B), fecolith (Figs 10.14A and B), bursa (Fig. 10.15), osteoarthritis (Figs 10.16A and B), synovial chondromatosis (Figs 10.17A and B), and in damaged tendons like tendon Achillis (Figs 10.18A and B).

Soft tissues calcification can be seen in some soft tissue tumors both benign and malignant. Arterial calcification is due to atheromatous change and is seen in the aortic arch abdominal aorta and iliacs frequent in the elderly. Wide spread arterial calcification may be seen in hyperparathyroidism. Other conditions with a high serum calcium such as chronic renal failure can give rise to calcification around joints. Scleroderma is associated with calcification in the digits. Gout shows calcified tophi in the soft tissues and dermatomyositis can give rise to calcification in the soft tissues.

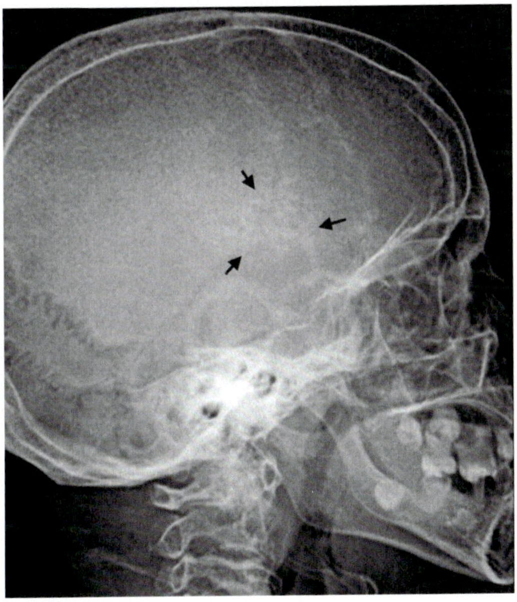

Fig. 10.10: X-ray of skull shows soft tissue calcification in a case of pseudohypoparathyroidism

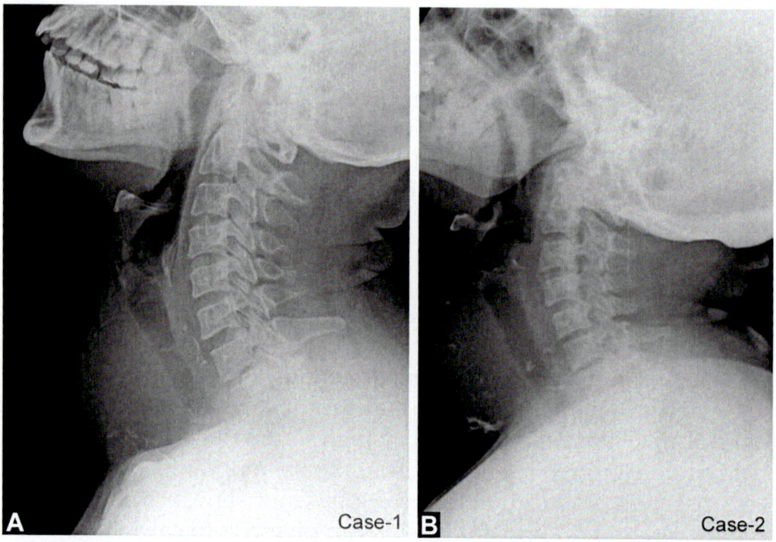


**Figs 10.11A and B:** X-ray for soft tissues of neck in two different cases show calcification in carcinoma of thyroid

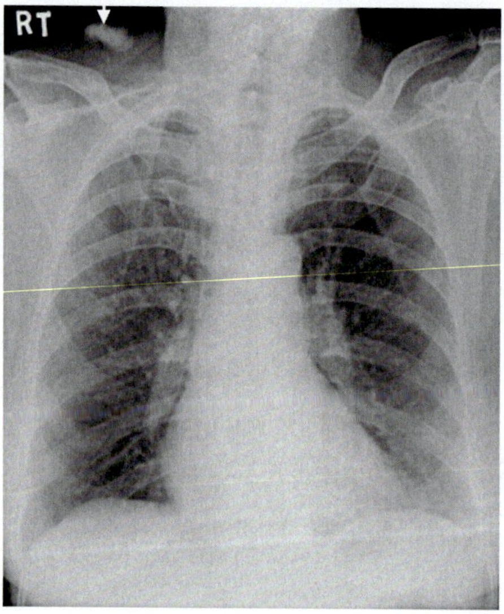


**Fig. 10.12:** X-ray of chest shows calcification in tuberculous cervical lymph nodes

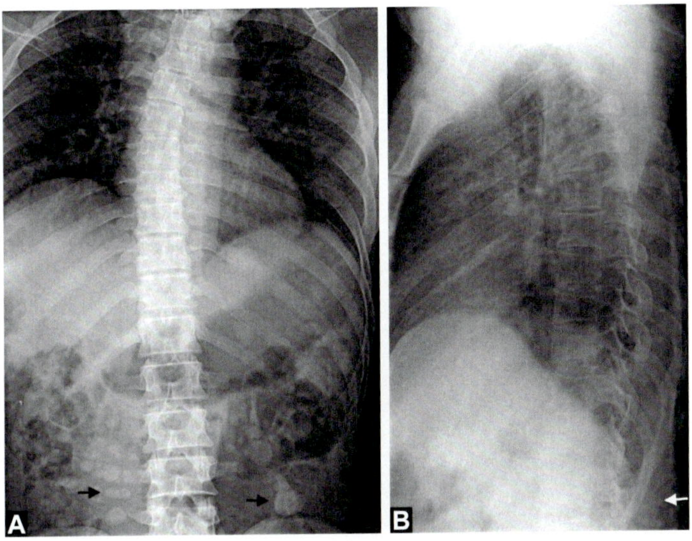

Figs 10.13A and B: X-rays of chest and abdomen show calcification in the wall in a case of abdominal neurofibromatosis

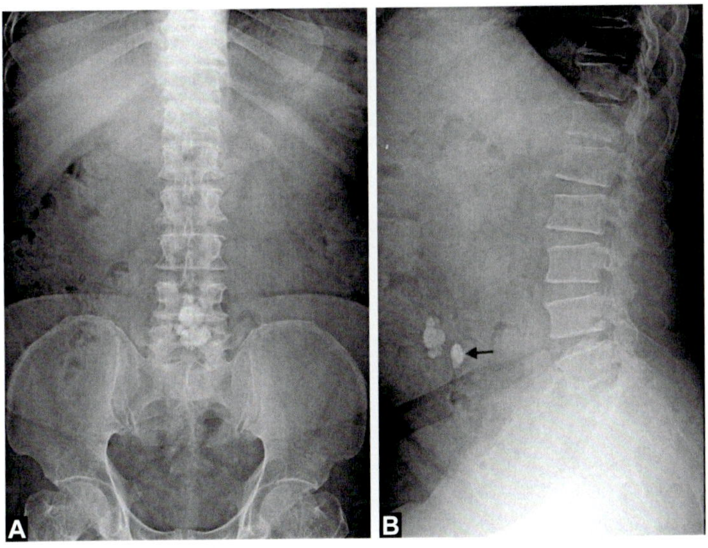

Figs 10.14A and B: X-rays of abdomen show well defined densities due to fecoliths

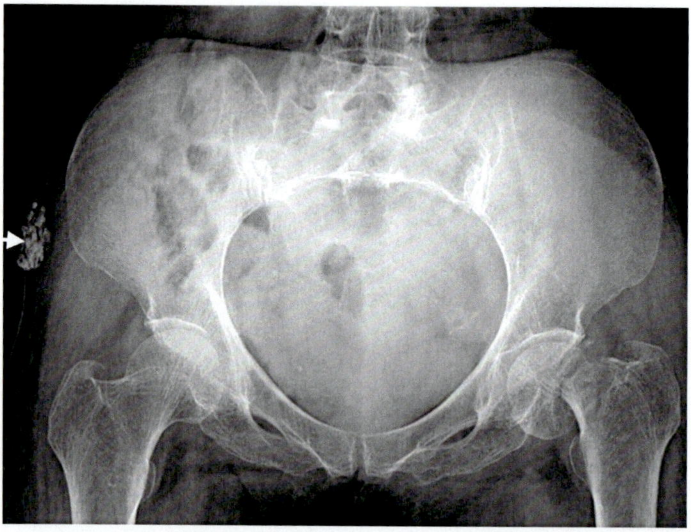

**Fig. 10.15:** X-ray of pelvis shows speckled calcification on right side in a bursa

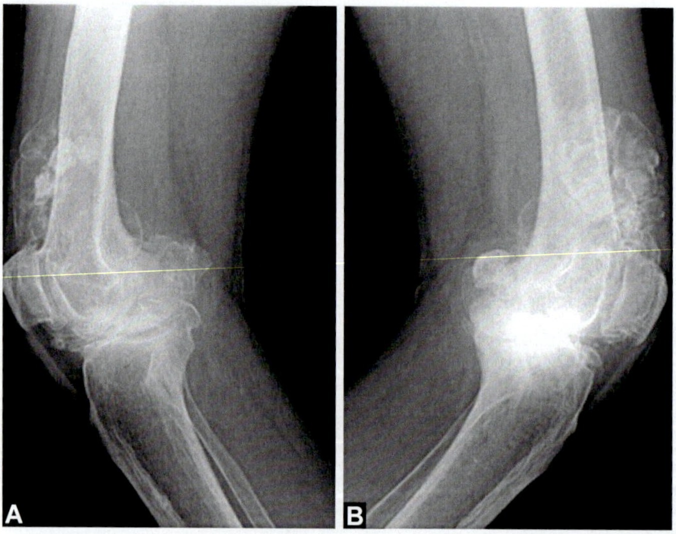


**Figs 10.16A and B:** X-rays of both knees show calcified loose bodies in a case of osteoarthritis

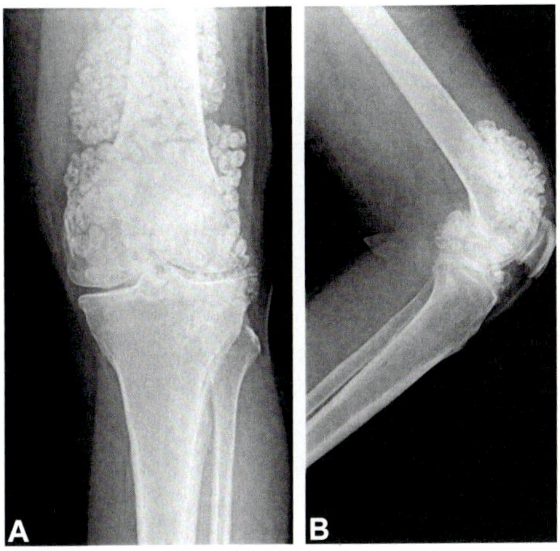


**Figs 10.17A and B:** X-ray of right knee: (A) AP; (B) lateral view show synovial chondromatosis

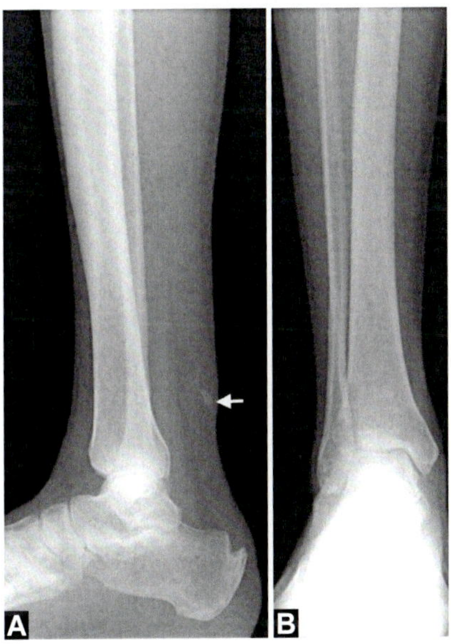


**Figs 10.18A and B:** X-rays of leg and ankle show calcification in a damaged tendo Achilles

## BREAST SCREENING

Breast cancer is the second most common malignancy after carcinoma cervix. Cancer is more common in nulliparous or woman with low parity. Sixty-six percent of breast cancers occur in women above the age of 50 years but can occur at any age after 20 years, 25% of patients with carcinoma have a positive family history and carcinoma tends to affect successive generations approximately 10 years earlier. Screening may detect cancers early, when they are treatable.

Screening methods to detect breast cancer include:

1. Education to the females for frequent self manual breast palpation for lump.
2. Clinical breast examination by clinician.
3. Mammography, thermography and occasionally MRI.

### *Digital Mammography*

High-quality digital mammography is the most effective technology presently available for breast cancer screening. Digital mammography is a mammography technique for recording X-ray images in computer code instead of on X-ray film, as with conventional mammography. Digital mammography leads to increased cancer detection rates. Digital mammography delivers significantly less radiation than conventional mammography.

Breast cancer screening should begin at the age of 40 years or earlier.

### Breast MRI

Breast MRI is not used for routine breast cancer screening, but clinical trials are being performed to determine if MRI is valuable for screening certain women, such as young women at high risk for breast cancer. MRI is also sometimes useful in imaging dense breast tissue, which is often seen in younger women and in viewing breast abnormalities that can be felt but are not visible with conventional mammography. Ultrasound is not modality for breast screening.

## CARCINOMA *IN SITU*

Carcinoma *in situ* (CIS) is an early form of carcinoma defined by the absence of invasion of surrounding tissues. It involves only the place in which it has begun and has not spread. It is an early-stage tumor. At CIS stage, there is no mass lesion and the lesion is flat or follows the existing architecture of the organ. CIS is considered a precursor or incipient form of cancer that may, if left untreated long enough, transform into a malignant neoplasm. Carcinoma *in situ* is synonymous with high-grade dysplasia in most organs. CIS is usually treated much the same way as a malignant tumor.

Common sites for CIS are bladder, cervix, prostate, ductal carcinoma *in situ* (DCIS) of the breast and Bowen's disease is squamous CIS of the skin

## LIPOMA

Lipoma is the most common benign tumor. It commonly occurs in head, neck, palm, sole and gastrointestinal tract. It can be localized or diffuse, single or multiple.

Sites of lipoma are subcutaneous, subfascial, intramuscular, intermuscular, periosteal, subserosal, submucosal, extradural and intra-articular.

Lipomas attain large size in thigh, shoulder, retroperitoneum and back. They present as localized, lobular, nontender and semifluctuant swelling. Submucosal lipoma can cause intestinal obstruction due to intussusceptions.

On plain film, it appears as a lucency in contrast with surrounding soft tissues. CT provides a definitive diagnosis of lipoma as the characteristic attenuation of fat is (-) 50 to (-) 200 HU (Hounsfield units). It also helps to localize the origin and to identify malignant degeneration of a benign lesion.

Complications are sarcomatous degeneration into liposarcoma, myxomatous degeneration, saponification and calcification.

# 11 CHAPTER Interventional Imaging

Chapter Outline

- Interventional Radiology
- CT Guided Precision Biopsy

## INTERVENTIONAL RADIOLOGY

The principle of interventional radiology (IR) is to diagnose or treat the disease using the least invasive technique. In IR, fluoroscopy, ultrasound, CT, and MRI are used to advance a catheter or probe into the body to diagnose or treat the disease. Images direct interventional procedures, which are usually done with needles and catheters. The images provide pathway that allow guiding the tools through the body to the area of pathology. This minimizes the trauma, reduce infection and grossly reduce recovery time.

Common IR procedures are:

1. Biopsy of a tissue sample from the area of interest is taken for pathological examination from a percutaneous approach.
2. In nephrostomy placement of a catheter directly into the kidney to drain urine in situations where normal flow of urine is obstructed. Through nephrostomy nephroureteral stents can be placed through the ureter and into the bladder.

3. In biliary intervention catheters are placed in the biliary system to bypass biliary obstructions for decompression of biliary system. Permanent biliary stents are also positioned.
4. In cholecystostomy tube is placed into the gallbladder to remove infected bile in patients with cholecystitis, who are too weak or too sick to undergo surgery.
5. In angiography the blood vessels are mapped to look for abnormalities with the use of iodinated contrast and gadolinium based agents.
6. In balloon angioplasty the narrow or blocked blood vessels are dilated using a balloon; followed by placement of self-expanding metallic stents.
7. In embolization abnormal blood vessels are blocked to stop bleeding. A variety of embolic agents are used, including alcohol, glue, metallic coils, poly-viny alcohol particles.
8. In thrombolysis the blood clots are dissolved with both pharmaceutical and mechanical means.
9. *In chemoembolization:* Cancer treatment is straight delivered to a tumor through its blood supply.
10. In radioembolization the radioactive microspheres are delivered to the tumor to kill the tumor cells while minimizing exposure to healthy cells.

A variety of catheters used in interventional radiology that include catheters, microcatheters, drainage catheters, balloon catheters and central venous catheters.

IR procedures are performed on an outpatient basis or may require a short hospital stay. General anesthesia generally is not required. Complications, pain and recovery time are substantially reduced and the procedures are less expensive than surgery.

Anterior mediastinal tumors like thymic cyst (Figs 11.1 and 11.2), thymic, lymphatic, or germ cell tumors are easily accessible to needle biopsy.

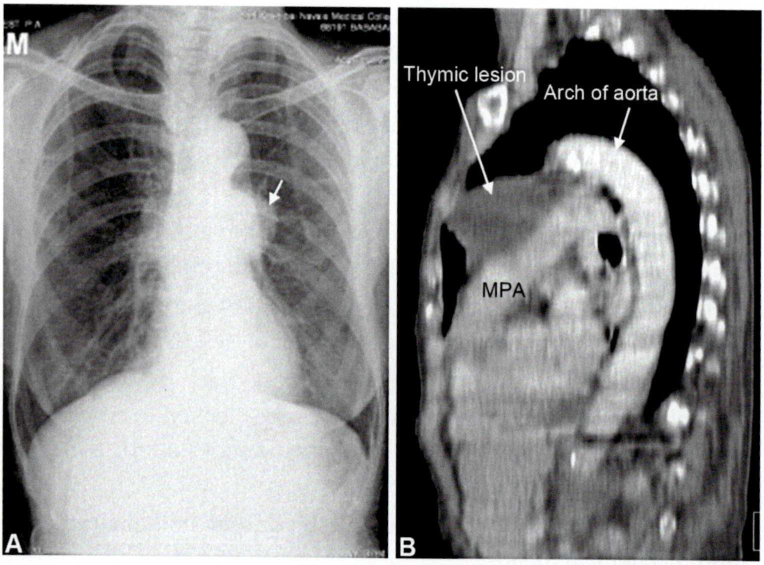


**Figs 11.1A and B:** (A) Chest X-ray of a 56 years old female shows anterior mediastinal left parahilar rounded opacity; (B) CT chest coronal reconstruction revealed a 4.4 X 5.8 cm well-defined unilocular cystic lesion (CT value 16 HU) in anterior mediastinum in the region of thymus on left side. The lesion had thin enhancing wall suggestive of thymic cyst. No evidence of calcification, mediastinal or hilar adenopathy was seen

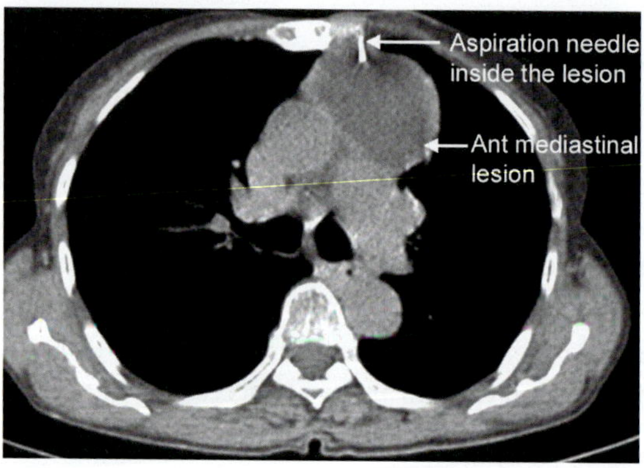


**Fig. 11.2:** Same case as Fig. 11.1, CT guided aspiration was done and 5 cc of brownish fluid (suggesting some hemorrhage) was aspirated and a diagnosis of thymic cyst was confirmed

## CT GUIDED PRECISION BIOPSY

CT guided precision robotic assistance biopsy with automated planner (Figs 11.3 to 11.5) reduce the number of needle passes, time spent and number of check scans which leads to significant reduction to patient's radiation dosage treated by this technique. Caroticocavernous and even vertebral AV fistula have also been treated with an ingenious detachable balloon introduced by percutaneous catheter. Dural AV fistula has also been successfully treated by embolization as have aneurysms.

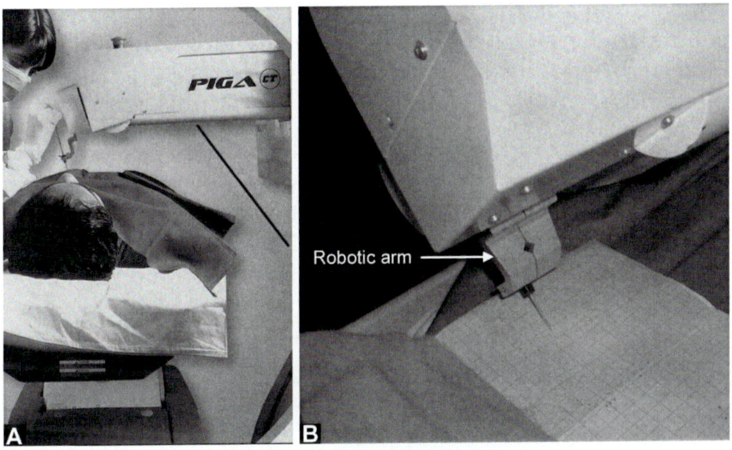


**Figs 11.3A and B:** (A) PIGA CT guided precision robotic assistance biopsy automated planner; (B) Magnified view of the robotic arm with biopsy needle

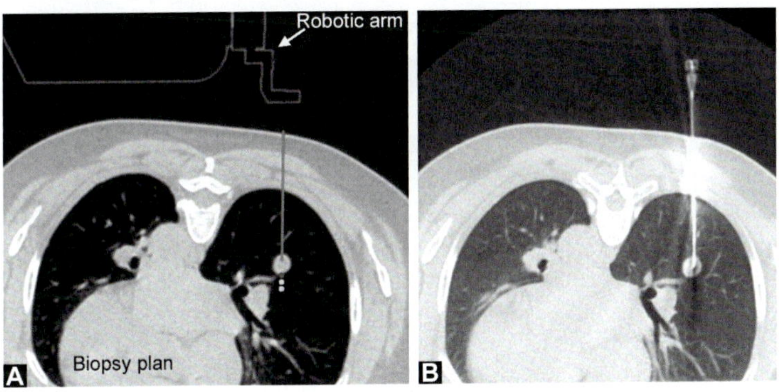


**Figs 11.4A and B:** (A) Plan for posterior straight approach biopsy (red line) for a 12 mm nodule in right lung; (B) Check scan shows precise positioning of needle in the nodule

**Percutaneous biliary duct drainage:** Patients with obstructive jaundice can be investigated by fine needle percutaneous cholangiography. Once the dilated ducts have been demonstrated these can also be catheterized percutaneously and a drain left *in situ* to decompress the biliary system and relieve the patient's acute symptoms.

**Percutaneous removal of biliary duct stones:** A major problem in the biliary tract is the patient with stones in the ducts which have not been found at operation and are later demonstrated by postoperative T-tube cholangiography. It is possible for the radiologist to remove such stones and save the patient from a further laparotomy. A guide wire is inserted into the ducts through the T-tube tract and a catheter with a wire snare is passed over the guide wire and into the ducts. The stones can then be snared and removed through the T-Tube tract.

**TIPS:** Transjugular intrahepatic portosystemic stent (TIPS) shunting is being increasingly used to create a portosystemic shunt between hepatic and portal vein branches in the treatment and control of complications in patients withportal hypertension. The interventional radiologist uses a percutaneous transjugular approach to the liver for a procedure which previously required major surgery.

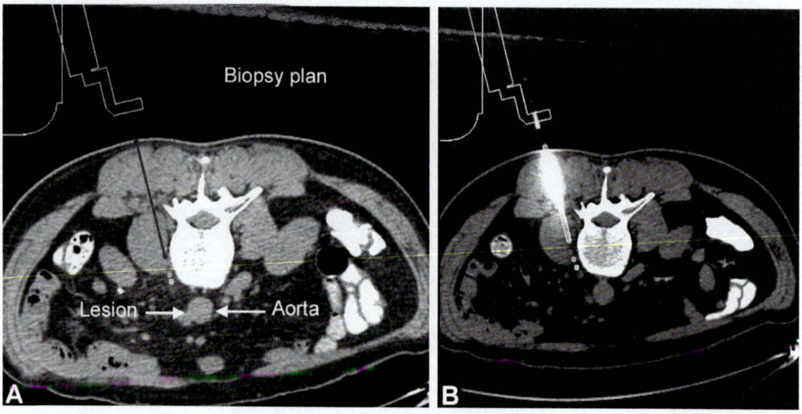


Figs 11.5A and B: (A) Posterior approach biopsy plan for a 9 mm left para-aortic lymph node; (B) The needle held in robotic arm is in the process of moving into the left para-aortic lymph node

# 12 CHAPTER

# Miscellaneous

**Chapter Outline**

- Production of X-rays
- Radiotherapy
- Physical Principle of CT Scan Imaging
- Radiation Safety Measures
- Endoscopic Ultrasonography
- Physical Principle of Magnetic Resonance Imaging
- Picture Archiving and Communication System
- Computed Radiography and Digital or Direct Radiography
- Ossification Centers

## PRODUCTION OF X-RAYS

X-rays are invisible, highly penetrating, electromagnetic radiations having wavelength of 0.1-1 Å (Armstrong) in the range of 0.01 to 10 nanometers and speed is same as that of light ($3 \times 10^8$ m/sec). They are considered as a form of modified electrons.

X-ray tube is a diode consisting of tungsten filament cathode and a rotating anode target of tungsten held in an evacuated glass. Tungsten anode is inclined at an angle so that it works on line-focus principle.

X-rays are produced when the electron beam strikes the anode made of tungsten or molybdenum. Tungsten (atomic number 74) is used as target material for X-ray production. Molybdenum (atomic number 42) is used as the target in mammography.

Cathode is connected to the negative terminal and consists of small coil of wire made of tungsten (filament). Cathode generates the electrons from the electric circuit and focuses them into well defined beam aimed at anode. Anode is relatively large piece of metal that connects to positive end of electric circuit. It converts electronic energy into X-rays and rapidly dissipates heat produced during this process. Anode is made up of tungsten because it has high melting point, low rate of evaporation and maintains strength at high temperature (Fig. 12.1).

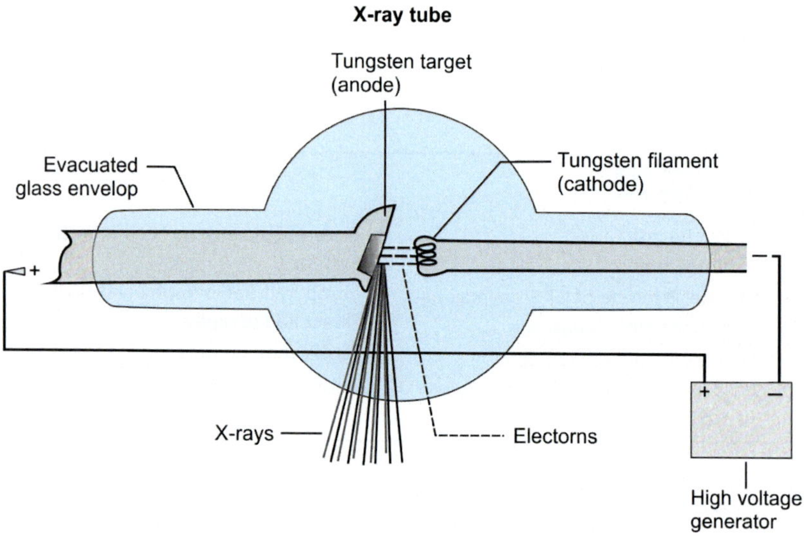


Fig. 12.1: Line diagram shows production of X-rays

The electrons are produced by cathode filament by electric current, emitting photo electrons. The electrons coming from the filament cathode are then accelerated towards the target anode by a large electrical potential applied between the filament and target. When the beam of electrons hits the target anode there is rapid deceleration of electrons leading to emission of X-rays and heat. About 1% of the energy generated is emitted as X-rays. The rest of the energy is released as heat.

The assembly of cathode and anode is enclosed in an envelope which is made of glass. It provides support and electric insulation, keeps cathode and anode in air tight enclosure and maintains vacuum in tube. Housing is the outermost covering that encloses and supports the envelope. It is filled with oil that provides electric insulation, allows heat dissipation and cooling.

Modern X-ray tubes are based on hot cathode tube principle invented by Coolidge in 1913 which enables excellent control of kVp (kilovolt peak) and mAs (milliampere second). kVp is responsible for penetration of X-ray beam, low kVp gives high contrast. mAs is responsible for the film blackening. The radiation intensity on the cathode side of the X-ray tube is higher than on the anode side and this principle is called as the Heel effect. The heat generated in the tube is dissipated in three ways: conduction, convection and radiation. Diagnostic X-ray machine uses voltage upto 150 kVp whereas machines used for radiotherapy use high voltage > 200 kV.

Two different interactions give rise to X-rays. An interaction with electron shell produce characteristic X-rays photons, while interaction with atomic nucleus produces Bremsstrahlung X-ray photons. In diagnostic radiology about 85% of X-rays arise from Bremsstrahlung radiation and 15% from characteristic radiation.

X-ray filter made of aluminum absorbs low energy radiation and decreases unnecessary patient exposure and thus improves film contrast. Grid is made of parallel lead lines with intervening radiolucent material. It absorbs scattered radiation. Cones and collimators restrict field size and decrease scatter.

Distance from X-ray tube (focus) to the X-ray film is called focus film distance (FFD). It is 100 cm for usual radiographs of extremities, abdomen and skull. However, for standing radiograph of chest it is 180 cm (6 ft) so as to reduce the magnification.

## RADIOTHERAPY

Radiotherapy is treatment of diseases by means of X-rays or other forms of radioactivity like alpha particles, gamma rays, electron, proton, neutron and positron.

### Modalities of Radiotherapy

Teletherapy is a form of treatment where a radioactive source is placed at a distance from the patient, i.e. external beam therapy. Cobalt-60 and linear accelerator are used for teletherapy. Three main types of radiation are used in the radiation therapy-Gamma rays, X-rays and Electron beam. Teletherapy has two broad subgroups depending on the beam quality and their use:

a. Kilovoltage therapy
b. Megavoltage therapy

Brachytherapy is radiation therapy where radioactive materials are placed in direct contact with the tissue being treated. Brachytherapy can be:

a. Interstitial: Radioactive sources are placed directly into the tumor in the form of needles
b. Intracavity: Containers that hold the radioactive sources are put into the body cavities.

Adverse effects of radiotherapy are given in Radiation Safety Measures under the sub heading Effects of Radiation.

## PHYSICAL PRINCIPLE OF CT SCAN IMAGING

CT was invented in 1972 by British engineer, Sir Godfrey Newbold Hounsfield in Hayes, United Kingdom at EMI Central Research Laboratories using X-rays. EMI laboratories is best known today for its music and recording business. About the same time South Africa-born American physicist, Allan McLeod Cormack of Tufts University in Massachusetts independently invented a similar process, and both shared the 1979 Nobel Prize.

The first clinical CT scan was installed in 1974. The initial systems were dedicated only to head scanning due to small gantry, but soon this was overcome and whole body CT system with larger gantry became available in 1976.

Basic principle is to obtain a tomogram having thickness in millimeters of the region of interest using pencil beam X-radiation. The radiation transmitted through the patient is counted by scintillation detector. This information when fed in the computer is analyzed by mathematical algorithms and reconstructed as a tomographic image by the computer so as to provide an insight into the structure being studied (Table 12.1).

### Developments in CT Technology

#### *Conventional Axial CT (Table 12.1)*

**Table 12.1:** Generations of CT scan

| Generation of CT scan | Motion of X-ray tube-detector system | Stationary detectors | X-ray beam type |
|---|---|---|---|
| First | Translate-Rotate | Two detectors | Pencil beam |
| Second | Translate-Rotate | Multiple detectors upto 30 | Narrow fan beam (10°) |
| Third | Rotate-Rotate | Multiple detectors upto 750 | Wide fan beam (50°) |
| Fourth | Rotate-Fixed | Ring of 1500-4500 detectors | Fan beam |

### Spiral/Helical CT

Spiral CT uses the conventional technology in conjunction with slip ring technology, which simultaneously provides high voltage for X-ray tube, low voltage for control unit and transmits digital data from detector array. Slip ring is a circular instrument with sliding bushes that enables the gantry to rotate continuously while the patient table moves into the gantry simultaneously, thus three-dimensional volume rendered image can be obtained. The advantages over the conventional scanner are the reduced scan time, reduced radiation exposure and reduced contrast requirement with superior information.

### Electron Beam CT (EBCT)

In EBCT, both the X-ray source and the detectors are stationary. High energy focused electron beam is magnetically steered on the tungsten target to emit X-rays which pass through the subject on to the detectors and image is acquired. EBCT is particularly used for faster imaging in cardiac studies.

### Multislice/Multidetector CT (MDCT)

Spiral CT uses single row of detectors, resulting in a single slice per gantry rotation. Multislice CT, multiple detector arrays are used resulting in multiple slices per gantry rotation. In addition, fan beam geometry of spiral CT is replaced by cone beam geometry.

The major advantages over spiral CT are improved spatial and temporal resolution, reduced image noise, faster and longer anatomic coverage and increased concentration of intravenous contrast.

### Dual Source CT

The dual energy technology of the new Flash CT provides higher contrast between normal and abnormal tissues making it easier to see abnormalities while reducing radiation. With its two rotating X-ray tubes, enhanced speed and power allows children to be screened more effectively. It turns off the radiation when it comes close to sensitive tissue areas of the body like thyroid, breasts, or eye lens.

Pediatric patients benefit because they do not need to hold breath or lay completely still during the examination and they do not have to be sedated.

## Hounsfield Units

CT numbers recognized by the computer are from (-) 1000 to (+) 1000, i.e. a range of 2000 Hounsfield units which are present in the image as 2000 shades of gray, but our eye cannot precisely discriminate between these 2000 different shades.

Hounsfield scale assigns attenuation value of water as zero (HU 0), and other tissues their attenuation value as compared to water as shown in Table 12.2.

**Table 12.2:** Attenuation value of various tissues on CT scan

| Tissue | Attenuation value in HU |
|---|---|
| Air | (-)1000 |
| Lung | (-) 400 to (-) 800 |
| Fat | (-) 40 to (-) 100 |
| Water | 0 |
| Fresh blood | 55 to 65 |
| Soft tissue | 40 to 80 |
| Bone | 400 to 1000 |

### *Window Level (WL) and Window Width (WW)*

To permit the viewer to understand the image, only a restricted number of HU are put on view and this is accomplished by setting the WL and WW on the console to a suitable range of Hounsfield units, depending on the tissue, for interpreting the image. The expression WL represents the central Hounsfield value of all the Hounsfield numbers within the WW. Tissues with CT numbers outside this array are shown as either black or white. Both the WL and WW can be set on the displayed image as desired by the viewer. On CT examination of the chest, a WW of 300 to 350 and WL of 35 to 45 are chosen to image the mediastinum (soft tissue window) whereas WW of 1500 and WL of 0 is used to assess the lung.

### *Image Reconstruction*

The acquisition of volumetric data using spiral CT means that the images can be postprocessed in ways appropriate to the clinical situation.

Multiplanar reformatting (MPR) is by taking standard axial images and subject to the three-dimensional array of CT numbers obtained with a series of contiguous slices; and can be viewed in sagittal, coronal, oblique and paraxial planes (Figs 12.2A to C).

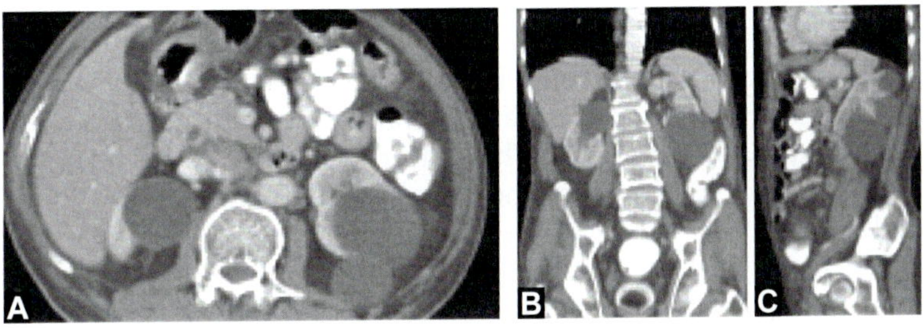

**Figs 12.2A to C:** Bilateral renal cysts seen in axial section (A) are reformatted into sagittal (B) and coronal (C) planes

## Three-Dimensional Imaging

Many fractures like fracture of the mandible associated with frontal bone with or without walls of sinuses can be reconstructed into a 3-dimensional image (Figs 12.3A to D).

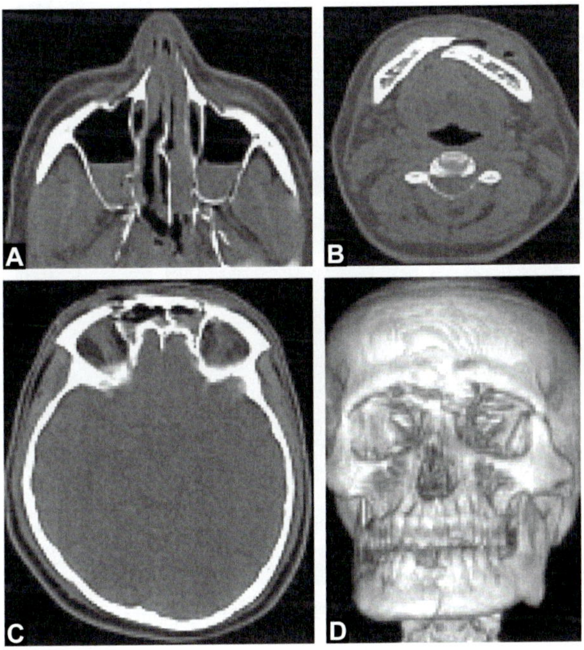

**Figs 12.3A to D:** Fracture of body of mandible and frontal bone. With bilateral maxillary hemosinus. D shows the 3D image of face including mandible

## CT Angiography

CT angiography (CTA) sequence is created subsequent to intravenous contrast, images are acquired in the arterial phase and then reconstructed and exhibited in 2D or 3D format. This performance is used for imaging the aorta, renal, cerebral, coronary and peripheral arteries (Figs 12.4A to F and 12.5, 12.6).

CT is readily available in most hospitals and stand-alone CT centers. It is fast imaging modality and provides with cross sectional high resolution images. Data acquired on axial scans can be used for multiplanar and 3D reconstructions. It detects subtle differences between body tissues. However it uses X-rays which have radiation hazards, CT need contrast media for enhanced soft tissue contrast. Contrast is contraindicated in asthma, cardiac disease, renal and certain thyroid conditions.

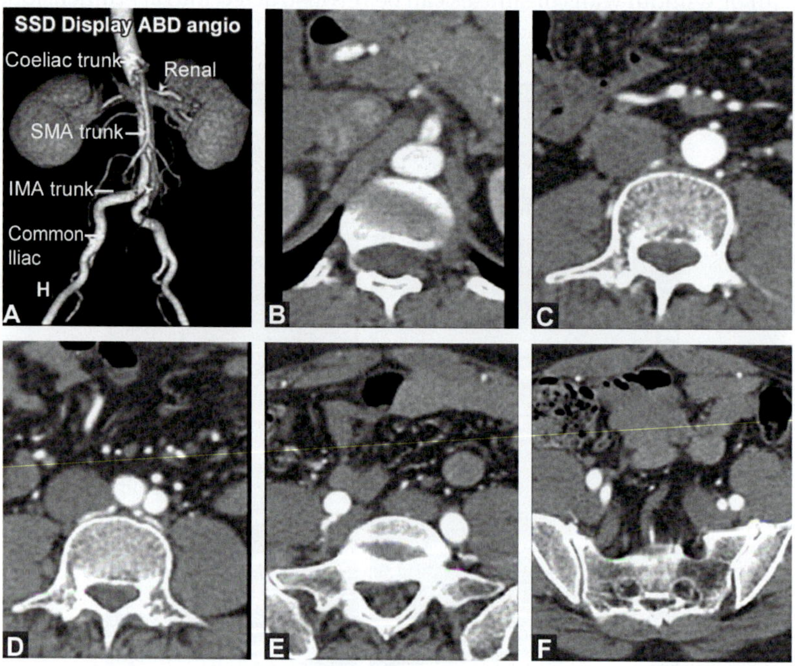


**Figs 12.4A to F:** CT abdominal angiography

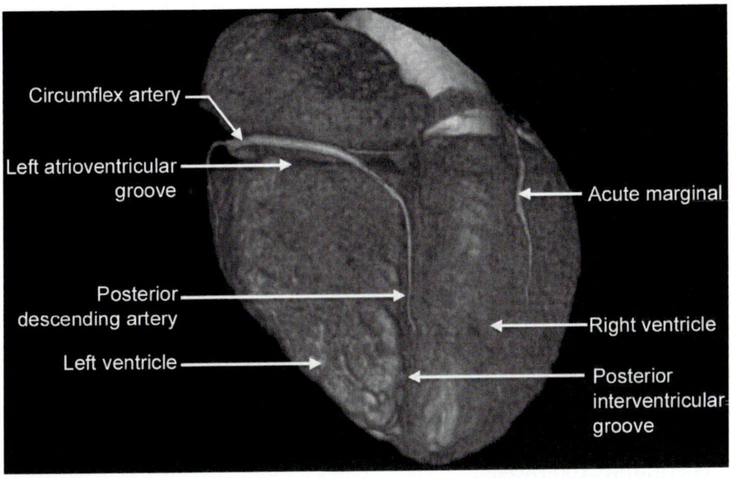


**Fig. 12.5:** Volume rendered image posterior coronal plane shows coronary arteries

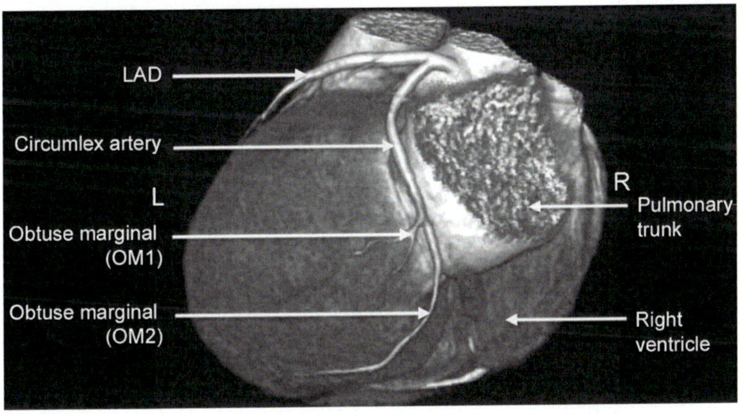


**Fig. 12.6:** Volume rendered image posterior oblique coronal plane shows coronary arteries

## RADIATION SAFETY MEASURES

Radiation is a form of energy which can travel from one place to another even in vacuum. Radiation hazards are the harmful effects that can occur to the body due to radiations.

Heat and light are forms of radiations that can be felt. Although X-rays are ionizing radiations, they cannot be felt by the skin. Hence, it is important to be aware of radiation hazards and radiation protection.

Natural sources of radiation are radon and cosmic rays. Artificial sources of radiation are:

a. Diagnostic radiation in the form of radiography, CT scan, PET scan and nuclear scan.
b. Therapeutic radiation in the form of brachytherapy and radiotherapy.

## Units of Radiation

As per the International System of Units, dose of ionizing radiation is measured in unit called as gray (Gy). One Gy is defined as that quantity of radiation which results in energy deposition of one Joule per kilogram in the irradiated tissue. Gray has replaced the earlier unit known as the rad. 1 Gy is equal to 100 rads.

Effective dose of radiation is different for different tissues and is measured in terms of a unit called as Sievert (Sv). This depends on the quality factor (Q) of the tissue which permits passage of energy. Dose equivalent (Sv) = Quality factor (Q) × Dose (Gy).

## Effects of Radiation

Stochastic effects of radiation are the ones whose probability of occurrence increases with increase in dose and include cancer and genetic effects. Deterministic effects are the ones which increase in severity with increase in dose and include cataract, blood dyscrasias and impaired fertility.

Irradiation in utero can lead to developmental abnormalities (8–25 weeks), cancer which can be expressed in childhood or in adults due to DNA damage by radiation. Preconception maternal irradiation in therapeutic doses gives rise to defects in 1 out of 10 exposed children. Nonurgent radiological testing should not be done between 8 and 17 weeks of gestation, which is the most sensitive period for organogenesis. Children are 10 times more sensitive to hazards of radiations than adults. Hence, radiography with high kV and low mAs technique is recommended in children.

Acute radiation syndrome is said to occur when high doses kill so many cells that tissues and organs are damaged immediately. The higher the radiation dose, the sooner the effects of radiation will appear and higher will be the probability of death. This was seen in atomic bomb survivors in 1945 and emergency workers responding to the 1986 Chernobyl nuclear power plant accident who received radiation to the tune of 800 to 16,000 mSv.

Acute radiation at doses in excess of 100 Gy to the total body, usually result in death within 24 to 48 hrs from neurological and cardiovascular failure. This is known as the cerebrovascular syndrome. Chronic radiation causes radiation pneumonitis and even permanent scarring that results in respiratory compromise.

### Average Effective Dose in Millisieverts (mSv)

**Table 12.3:** Average effective dose in millisieverts (mSv)

| S. No. | Examination | Radiation Dose |
|---|---|---|
| 1. | X-ray Chest | 0.02 |
| 2. | CT Orbits | 0.8 |
| 3. | CT Temporal bone | 1.0 |
| 4. | CT Head | 2.0 |
| 5. | CT Spine | 3.0 |
| 6. | CT Chest | 8.0 |
| 7. | CT Abdomen | 10.0 |
| 8. | CT Pelvis | 10.0 |

The International Commission of Radiation Protection (ICRP) was formed in 1928 on the recommendation of the first International Congress of Radiology in 1925 which formed the International Commission on Radiation Units (ICRU). The National Commission for Radiation Protection (NCRP) in America and the Atomic Energy Regulatory Board (AERB) in India are the regulatory bodies that recommend norms for permissible doses of radiation for radiation workers and for the general public.

Atomic Energy Regulatory Board (AERB) which is the Indian Regulatory Board was constituted on November 15, 1983 by the President of India by exercising the powers conferred by Section 27 of the Atomic Energy Act, 1962. The Regulatory Authority of AERB is derived from the rules and notifications promulgated under the Atomic Energy Act, 1962 and the Environmental (Protection) Act, 1986. Radiation safety in handling of radiation generating equipment is governed by Section 17 of the Atomic Energy Act, 1962 and the Radiation Protection Rules, 1971 issued under the Act.

The overall objective of radiation protection is to provide an appropriate standard of protection for man without unduly limiting the beneficial practices giving rise to radiation exposure.

Atomic Energy Regulatory Board (AERB) recommends and lays down guidelines regarding the specifications of medical X-ray equipment, for the room layout of X-ray installation, regarding the work practices in X-ray department, the protective devices and also the responsibilities of the radiation personnel, employer and Radiation Safety Officer (RSO). It is the authority in India which exercises a regulatory control and has the power to decommissioning X-ray installations and also for imposing penalties on any person contravening these rules.

## Benefit Risk Analysis

Since radiation exposure entails inherent risks of radiation effects, no decision to expose an individual can be undertaken without weighing benefits of exposure against potential risks that is, making a benefit risk analysis.

## Principles of Radiation Protection

1. Justification of a practice
2. Optimized protection
3. Dose limitation

## Radiation Protection Actions

The triad of radiation protection actions comprise of "time distance-shielding". Reduction of exposure time, increasing distance from source, shielding of patients and occupational workers, have proven to be of great importance.

## Shielding

Shielding implies that certain materials (concrete, lead) will attenuate radiation (reduce its intensity) when they are placed between the source of radiation and the exposed individual.

## Source Shielding

X-ray tube housing is lined with thin sheets of lead because X-rays produced in the tube are scattered in all directions, to protect both patients and personnel from leakage of radiation. AERB recommends a maximum allowable leakage radiation from tube housing not greater than 1 mGy per hour per 100 $cm^2$.

## Structural Shielding

The lead lined walls of radiology department are referred to as protective barriers because they are designed to protect individuals located outside the X-ray rooms from unwanted radiation.

1. Primary barrier is one which is directly struck by the primary or the useful beam.
2. Secondary barrier is one which is exposed to secondary radiation either by leakage from X-ray tube or by scattered radiation from the patient. The room housing X-ray unit should not be less than 18 $m^2$ for general purpose radiography and conventional fluoroscopy equipment and that of the CT room housing the gantry of the CT unit should not be less than 25 $m^2$.

Wall of the X-ray rooms on which primary X-ray beam falls should not be less than 35 cm thick brick or equivalent. Walls of the X-ray room on which scattered X-rays fall should not be less than 23 cm thick brick or equivalent. The walls and viewing window of the control booth should have material of 1.5 mm lead equivalent.

### Personnel Shielding

Shielding apparel should be used as and when necessary which comprise of lead aprons, eye glasses with side shields, hand gloves and thyroid shields. The minimum thickness of lead equivalent in the protective apparel should be 0.5 mm. These are classified as a secondary barrier to the effects of ionizing radiation as they protect an individual only from secondary (scattered) radiation and not the primary beam.

### Patient Shielding

Thyroid, breast and gonads are shielded to protect these organs especially in children and young adults. The responsibility for establishing a Radiation Protection Program rests with the hospital administration/owners of the X-ray facility. The administration is expected to appoint a Radiation Safety Committee (RSC) and a Radiation Safety Officer (RSO).

Every radiation worker prior to commencing radiation work and at subsequent intervals not exceeding 12 months shall be subjected to the medical examination.

### Radiation

Radiation Safety Officer (RSO) should be an individual with extensive training and education in areas such as radiation protection, radiation physics, radiation biology, instrumentation, dosimetry and shielding design. Duties include assisting the employer in meeting the relevant regulatory requirements applicable to the X-ray installation and ensuring that all radiation measuring and monitoring instruments under custody are properly calibrated and maintained in good condition.

## Recommended Dose Limits

Once pregnancy is established the dose equivalent to the surface of pregnant woman's abdomen should not exceed 2 mSv for the remainder of the pregnancy. Ten Day Rule states that all females of reproductive age who need an X-ray examination should get it done within first 10 days of menses to avoid irradiation to possible conception.

As a general principle radiation exposure (Table 12.3) should be less than 20 mSv/year for radiation workers and less than 1 mSv/year for general public. Optimization of protection can be achieved by optimizing the procedure to administer a radiation dose which is As Low As Reasonably Achievable (ALARA), so as to derive maximum diagnostic information with minimum discomfort to the patient.

## Detection of Radiation

Following are the methods of detecting radiation, based on physical and chemical effects produced by radiation exposure:

1. Ionization: The ability of radiation to produce ionization in air is the basis for radiation detection by the ionization chamber.
2. Photographic effect: The ability of radiation to blacken photographic film is the basis of detectors that use film.
3. Luminescence: When radiation strikes certain materials they emit light that is proportional to the radiation intensity.
4. Scintillation: Here radiation is converted into light, which is then directed to a photomultiplier tube, which then converts the light into an electrical pulse.

Personnel dosimetry is the monitoring of individuals who are exposed to radiation during the course of their work. It is accomplished through the use of devices such as the pocket dosimeter, the film badge or the thermoluminescent dosimeter (TLD). The dose is subsequently stated as an estimate of the effective dose equivalent to the whole body in mSv for the reporting period. Dosimeters used for personnel monitoring have dose measurement limit of 0.1–0.2 mSv (10–20 mrem).

Thermoluminescent dosimeter can measure exposures as low as 1.3 µC/kg (5 mR) and the pocket dosimeter can measure up to 50 µC/kg (200 mR). The film badge however cannot measure exposures < 2.6 µC/kg (10 mR). TLD can withstand certain degree of heat, humidity and pressure; their crystals are reusable and instantaneous readings are possible if the department has a TLD analyzer. The greatest disadvantage of a TLD is its cost.

## Ultrasonography

Diagnostic ultrasound is a noninvasive imaging modality utilizing high frequency sound energy in the range of 3 to 15 megahertz (MHz). This is well above the normal human ear response to sound frequency of 20-20,000 Hz.

Ultrasonography (USG) works on piezoelectric effect of crystals made from lead zirconate titanate or polyvinylidene difluoride and is used in forming images by using pulse echo principle. Gray scale (B) mode is used in general imaging. Motion (M) mode is used for echocardiography. Color Doppler ultrasound is used for imaging of vessels; Christian Doppler was first to put forth the principle of Doppler.

High frequency sound waves travel through human tissue; they are reflected on traversing interfaces. A transducer which emits high frequency sound is moved over the patient; the reflected waves are returned to the transducer resulting in an image by the computer.

Echoes or reflections of the ultrasound beam form interfaces between tissues with different acoustic properties, resulting in information on the size, shape and structure of organ or mass. Ultrasound is largely reflected by air-soft tissue interface and bone-soft tissue interface, thus being of relatively limited use in the chest and musculoskeletal system.

Ultrasonography does not use X-rays, as a result there is no risk of ionizing radiations. It is real time, permits multiplanar imaging, helps positive decision for a lesion to be cystic or solid. It is used to perform interventional procedures. The equipment is portable, inexpensive, easily available and low risk. It is low cost, being cheaper than other cross-sectional imaging techniques. Doppler evaluation allows analysis of blood flow. There are no known harmful effects of high frequency sound waves on human body.

Disadvantages of USG are few. It is difficult in obese patients and in viewing deep structures; it does not show function of tissues. Air, bone and fat are enemies to good ultrasound imaging.

Doppler ultrasonography employs the frequency shift in the reflected ultrasonic beam to recognize the moving fluid in the body. It demonstrates the presence and direction of blood flow. It gives red color coding for blood flowing towards the transducer and blue coding to blood flowing away from the transducer (Fig. 12.7). Doppler can be used to attain spectral trace that shows velocity of flow.

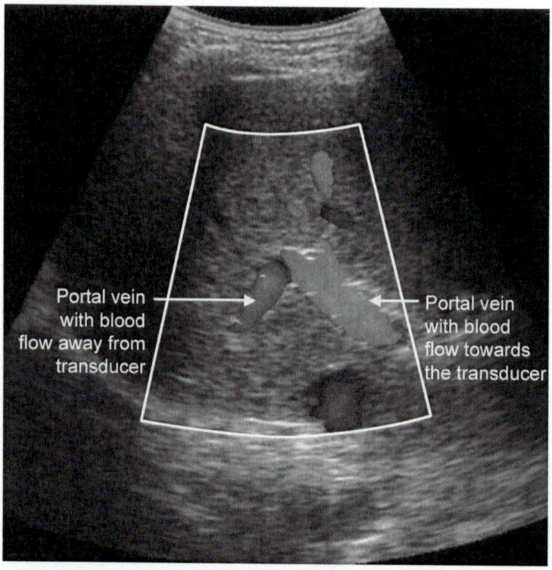


Fig. 12.7: Liver image, a Doppler interrogation box placed over the portal vein

## ENDOSCOPIC ULTRASONOGRAPHY

Endoscopic ultrasonography (EUS) utilizes the combined technology of videoendoscopy and high frequency ultrasound (US). US transducers (probes) used are either radial array or linear array. The frequency range is 7.5 to 12 MHz. The ultrasound endoprobe measures 13 mm in diameter. The system is forward oblique viewing and has water filled balloon to provide mucosal contact. A narrower blind scope is also available which relies on ultrasound for guidance and can be passed over a guide-wire so it is used when a stricture prevents the passage of the larger videoscope.

It allows visualization of five layers of walls of gastrointestinal tract. Disruption of the tissue planes delineated by these boundary echoes is vital to the diagnosis and staging of tumors.

### *Applications*

1. Esophagus and stomach for local tumor staging (T staging). Evaluation of regional lymph nodes within limited field of view.
2. Rectal endoscopic ultrasonography with a 360° rotating endoprobes is used to obtain high resolution images of the rectal wall and is used primarily to stage tumors.

3. Anal endosonography uses a modified rectal endoprobe to image the anal spincters, providing information about spincter integrity and morphology in patients who are anally incontinent.
4. Biliary tree endosonography has a developing role in the evaluation of the bile duct tumors at the ampulla or liver hilum to determine their operability. It also provides survey of common duct for bile duct stones and submucosal pathologies invisible to conventional endoscopy.

## PHYSICAL PRINCIPLE OF MAGNETIC RESONANCE IMAGING

Magnetic resonance imaging (MRI) is based on the principle of electromagnetic character of atomic nuclei which was first described by physicist Felix Bloch and Edward Purcell in 1946. They received a Noble prize for this in 1952. However, it was long after this that nuclear magnetic resonance was used for imaging. In 1973, Lauterbur showed that images of human body could be acquired by placing a magnetic field around it. First human images were published by Damadian et al in 1977. Since then use of MRI for medical imaging has seen an exponential growth and now it is a mainstay in the field of medical diagnostics.

Electromagnetism is at the core of MRI physics. When current is passed through a wire, a magnetic field is created around it. Similarly, in a nucleus with odd number of protons or neutrons, the electrons rotating around the nucleus produce a field around them. This gives a "charge" to the nucleus, also called as the spinning charge or "the spin". Thus these nuclei behave as tiny magnets. Hydrogen proton is the most favorable nucleus for MRI as it is widely available in the water molecules present in the body.

When these nuclei are placed in an external magnetic field ($B_0$), they either align along the magnetic field or against it. When the number of nuclei along the magnetic field is more as compared to those against the field, a net magnetization is created in the direction of the field.

In order to generate a signal from these spinning nuclei they have to be tipped out of alignment with $B_0$ (i.e. out of the longitudinal plane and towards the transverse plane). The signal generated by each rotating nucleus is much stronger if the nuclei precess in unison with each other at 90 degrees to the main magnetic field. For this a second magnetic field is introduced and it is referred to as $B_1$. This $B_1$ should be applied perpendicular to $B_0$, and it has to be at the resonant frequency. Radiofrequency (RF) coils are used to transmit $B_1$. If sufficient RF pulse is applied the spins are flipped into the transverse plane. This is the 90° RF pulse and it generates the strongest signal. However, as this is a high energy state, the signal starts decaying quickly and is called free induction decay (FID). This decay or relaxation is of two types:

T1 relaxation is the relaxation in the longitudinal plane due to the spins returning to the normal equilibrium state and aligning with the main magnetic field. In T2 relaxation there is dephasing in the transverse plane (90 degree plane). Each individual proton precesses at slightly different speed. After a while, the signal from protons in transverse plane degenerates as protons start precessing out of phase with each other. This is T2 relaxation.

In human tissue T1 is usually 10 times longer than T2 which means that T2 decay occurs before T1 recovery. In actual practice the T2 dephasing time is much quicker than the 'natural' T2 due to inhomogenities in the magnetic field $B_0$. This reduced T2 is called T2*.

T1W and T2W images result by manipulating the manner and frequency in which RF pulses are applied (Repetition to Time), and by changing time to start signal acquisition after RF has been applied (Time to Echo), T1-weighted or T2-weighted images can be obtained.

## Pulse Sequences

### *Partial saturation (PS)*

It is also known as gradient echo or field echo and it uses a 90° RF pulse.

### *Spin echo (SE)*

A 90° pulse is followed by 180° refocusing RF pulse.

### *Inversion recovery (IR)*

180° pulse is followed by a 90° pulse.

In a typical image acquisition, the basic unit of each sequence (i.e. the 90°-180° signal detection) is repeated hundreds of times. By altering the time to echo (TE) or time to repetition (TR), i.e. the time between successive 90° pulses, the signal contrast can be altered or weighted (Table 12.4). For example, if a long TE is used, inherent differences in T2 times of tissues will become apparent. Tissues with a long T2 (e.g. water) will take longer to decay and their signal will be greater (or appear brighter in the image) than the signal from tissue with a short T2 (e.g. fat). In a similar manner TR governs T1 contrast. Tissue, with a long TR (water) will take a long time to recover back to the equilibrium magnetization value, therefore, a short TR interval will make this tissue appear dark (Table 12.5) compared to tissue with a short T1 (fat). When TE and TR are chosen to minimize both these weightings, the signal contrast is only derived from the number or density of spins in a given tissue. This image is said to be proton density weighted (PDW).

Air is black in all sequences because of very few protons and cortical bone is always black due to no mobility of protons.

Each volume element in the body has a different resonant frequency which depends on the protons present within it. This produces a signal which is specific to the resonant frequency of that volume element. This signal is analyzed by the computers using a mathematical technique called as Fourier analysis.

Magnet forms the main component of the MRI, it is of two types:

1. Permanent or resistive magnets used in low field scanners and are usually referred to as open MRI,
2. Superconducting magnets are used in all scanners above 1.0 Tesla. It is wound from an alloy usually Niobium and Titanium (Nb-Ti) that has zero electrical resistance below a critical temperature. To maintain this temperature the magnet is enclosed and cooled by a cryogen containing liquid helium which has to be topped-up on a regular basis.

RF coils are needed to transmit and/or receive the MR signal. The RF coil should cover only the volume of interest. This gives an optimal signal-to-noise ratio (SNR). To achieve this there are various types of RF coils with trade-offs in terms of coverage and sensitivity, e.g. head coil being smaller in size provides better SNR. Body coil is integrated into the scanner bore and is not seen by the patient. Both these coils act as transceivers, i.e. they transmit and receive. Surface coils are used for imaging anatomy near to the coil. They are simple loop designs and have excellent SNR close to the coil but the sensitivity drops off rapidly with distance from the coil. These are only used as receivers, the body coil acting as the transmitter. Quadrature or circularly-polarized coils comprise of two coils 90° apart to improve SNR by a factor of 2½.

Advanced applications include diffusion imaging, perfusion imaging, functional MRI, spectroscopy, interventional MRI.

Possible adverse effects of MRI can be due to static magnetic field, gradients, RF heating, noise and claustrophobia.

Caution needs to be exercised while selecting patients for MRI. Patients with pacemakers, metallic implants, aneurysm clips should be excluded. Metallic objects should not be taken near the magnet as they can be injurious to the patient, personnel and equipment.

## Special Sequences

### *Short Tau Inversion Recovery (STIR) Sequence*

It is heavily T2-weighted imaging, as a result the fluid and edema return high signal intensity and it annuls out the signal from fat. The resultant images show the areas of pathology clearly. The sequence is useful in musculoskeletal imaging as it annuls the signal from normal fatty bone marrow.

### *Fluid Attenuated Inversion Recovery (FLAIR)*

This is an inversion-recovery pulse sequence that suppresses or annuls out the signal from fluid/CSF. The sequence is useful to show subtle lesions in the brain and spinal cord as it annuls the signal from CSF. It is useful to bring out the periventricular hyperintense lesions, e.g. in multiple sclerosis.

**Table 12.4:** Time to echo and time to repetition for MR sequences

| | Time to Echo TE | Time to Repetition TR |
|---|---|---|
| T1 weighted or T1W | Short TE | Short TR |
| T2 weighted or T2W | Long TE | Long TR |
| Proton density weighted or PDW | Short TE | Long TR |

**Table 12.5:** Signal intensity of various tissues at T1, T2 and proton density imaging

| Tissue | T1 | T2 | Proton Density |
|---|---|---|---|
| Fat | Bright | Bright (less than T1) | Bright |
| Water | Dark | Bright | Intermediate bright |
| Cerebral gray matter | Gray | Gray | Gray |
| Cerebral white matter | White | Dark | Dark |
| TR values | TR < 500 | TR > 1500 | TR > 1500 |
| TE values | TE 50 to 100 | TE > 80 | TE < 50 |

## Gradient Echo Sequence

This sequence reduces the scan times. This is achieved by giving a shorter RF pulse leading to a lesser amount of disruption to the magnetic vectors. The sequence is useful in identifying calcification and blood degradation products.

### Diffusion-Weighted Imaging

'Diffusion' portrays the movement of molecules due to random motion. It enables to distinguish between rapid diffusion of protons (unrestricted diffusion) and slow diffusion of protons (restricted diffusion). GRE pulse sequence has been devised to image the diffusion of water through tissues. It is a sensitive way of detecting acute brain infarcts, where diffusion is reduced or restricted.

### MR Angiography

The most common MR angiographic techniques are time-of-flight imaging and phase contrast. In these sequences, multiple RF pulses are applied with short TRs saturate the spins in stationary tissues. This results in suppression of the signal from stationary tissues in the imaging slab. In-flowing blood is unaffected by the repetitive RF pulses, as a result, as it enters the imaging slab, its signal is not suppressed and appears hyperintense compared with that of stationary tissue. Time-of-flight imaging may be 2D, with section-by-section acquisition, or 3D, with acquisition of a larger volume. Dynamic MRA can also be performed with intravenous gadolinium when in the vascular phase of enhancement.

## PICTURE ARCHIVING AND COMMUNICATION SYSTEM

Picture archiving and communication system (PACS), is based on universal DICOM (Digital imaging and communications in medicine) format. DICOM solutions are capable of storing and retrieving multi modality images in a proficient and secure manner in assisting and improving hospital workflow and patient diagnosis.

The aim of PACS is to replace conventional radiographs and reports with a completely electronic network, these digital images can be viewed on monitors in the radiology department, emergency rooms, inpatient and outpatient departments, thus saving time, improving efficiency of hospital and avoid recurring cost of hard copy images in a busy hospital. The three basic means of rendering plain radiographs images to digital are computed radiography (CR) using photostimulable phosphor plate technology; direct digital radiography (DDR) and digitizing conventional analog films. Nonimage data, such as scanned documents like PDF (portable document format) is also incorporated in DICOM format. Dictation of reports can be integrated into the system. The recording is automatically sent to a transcript writer's workstation for typing, but it can also be made available for access by physicians, avoiding typing delays for urgent results.

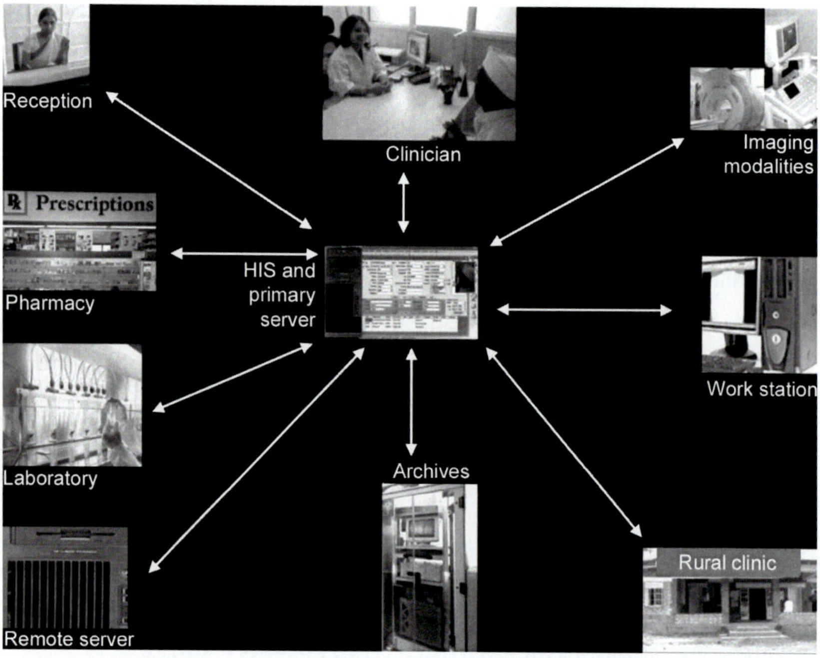


Fig. 12.8: Picture Archiving and Communication System (PACS) Flow chart

Radiology has led the way in developing PACS to its present high standards. PACS consists of four major components: the imaging modalities such as radiography, computed radiography, endoscopy, mammography, ultrasound, CT, PET-CT and MRI, a secured network for the transmission of patient information, workstations for interpreting and reviewing images and archives for the storage and retrieval of images and reports (Fig. 12.8). Backup copies of patient images are provisioned in case the image is lost from the PACS. There are several methods for backup storage of images, but they typically involve automatically sending copies of the images to a separate computer for storage, preferably off-site.

In PACS no patient is irradiated simply because a previous radiograph or CT scan has been lost; the image once acquired onto the PACS is always available when needed. Simultaneous multilocation viewing of the same image is possible on any workstation connected to the PACS. Numerous post processing soft copy manipulations are possible on the viewing monitor. Film packets are no longer an issue as PACS provides a filmless solution for all images. PACS can be integrated into the local area network and images from remote villages can be sent to the tertiary hospital for reporting.

PACS is an expensive investment initially but the costs can be recovered over a 5 years period. It requires a dedicated maintenance. It is important to train the doctors, technicians, nurses and other staff to use PACS effectively. Once PACS is fully operational no films are issued to patients.

PACS breaks the physical and time barriers associated with traditional film-based image retrieval, distribution and display. PACS can be linked to the internet, leading to teleradiology, the advantages of which are that images can be reviewed from home when on call, can provide linkage between two or more hospitals, outsourcing of imaging examinations in understaffed hospitals. PACS is offered by all the major medical imaging equipment manufacturers, medical IT companies and many independent software companies.

## COMPUTED RADIOGRAPHY AND DIGITAL OR DIRECT RADIOGRAPHY

Computed Radiography (CR) uses very equipment similar to conventional radiography except that in place of a X-ray film to create the image, an imaging plate (IP) made of photostimulable phosphor is used. The IP is positioned in a special cassette and placed under the body part or object to be examined and the X-ray exposure is made. Hence, instead of taking an exposed film to the darkroom for developing in chemical tanks or an automatic film processor, the IP is run through a special laser scanner or CR reader that reads and digitizes the image. The digital image can then be viewed and enhanced using software functions similar to other conventional digital image-processing software.

### Imaging Plate

The CR, IP contains photostimulable storage phosphors, which store the radiation level received at each point in local electron energies. When the plate is put through the scanner, the scanning laser beam causes the electrons to relax to lower energy levels, emitting light that is detected by a photo-multiplier tube, which is then converted to an electronic signal. The electronic signal is converted to discrete digital values and placed into the image pixel map to convert into visible diagnostic image. The laser scanners automatically erase the IP after laser scanning is complete. The IP can then be reused. Reusable phosphor plates are environmentally safe of radiations.

### Difference between Computed Radiography (CR) and Digital or Direct Radiography (DR)

Computed radiography (CR) and Digital or Direct radiography (DR) have many similarities. Both CR and DR use a medium to capture X-ray energy and both produce a digital image. Both CR and DR present an image within seconds of exposure. CR generally involves the use of a cassette that houses the IP, similar to traditional film-screen cassette, to record the image whereas DR captures the image directly onto a flat panel detector without the use of a cassette. Image enhancement can be applied to both CR and DR images in digital format.

CR system is reliable and is low cost conversion of multiple X-ray equipments into digital format. DR systems generally mean a full X-ray room replacements tied to a single X-ray generator. CR IPs can be retrofitted to existing exam rooms and used in multiple X-ray sites since IPs are processed through a CR reader (scanner) that can be shared between multiple exam rooms.

Advantages of CR or DR over convention X-rays

1. No silver based film or chemicals are required to process the films.
2. Images are available for digital view.
3. There are fewer retakes which results in lower overall dose to the patient.
4. Image acquisition is faster with immediate image previews availability.
5. Images can be enhanced digitally to aid interpretation.
6. Images can be stored on disk or transmitted for off site review.
7. Ever growing CR technology is affordable and cheaper than conventional radiographic operations.

## OSSIFICATION CENTERS (TABLES 12.6 TO 12.11, FIGURES 12.9 TO 12.14)

**Table 12.6:** Shoulder joint

| Bones | Ossification | |
|---|---|---|
| Body of scapula | 8th week of fetal life | |
| Body of clavicle (two centers) | 5th and 6th week of fetal life | |
| Shaft of humerus | 8th week of fetal life | |
| **Epiphysis** | **Appearance** | **Fusion** |
| Head of humerus | 1 year | |
| Greater tuberosity | 3 years | |
| Lesser tuberosity | 5 years | |
| Acromion process | 15–18 years | 25th year |
| Middle of coracoid process | 1 year | 15th year |
| Root of coracoid process | 17th year | 25th year |

*Contd...*

*Contd...*

| | | |
|---|---|---|
| Inferior angle of scapula | 14–20 years | 22–25 years |
| Medial border of scapula | 14–20 years | 22–25 years |
| Medial end of clavicle | 18–20 years | 25th year |

**Table 12.7:** Elbow joint

| **Bones** | **Ossification** | |
|---|---|---|
| Radial shaft | 8th week of fetal life | |
| Ulnar shaft | 8th week of fetal life | |
| **Epiphysis** | **Appearance** | **Fusion** |
| Lateral epicondyle | 10–12 years | 17–18 years |
| Medial epicondyle | 05–08 years | 17–18 years |
| Capitellum | 01–03 years | 17–18 years |
| Head of radius | 05–06 years | 16–19 years |
| Trochlea | 11th year | 18th year |
| Olecranon process | 10–13 years | 16–20 years |

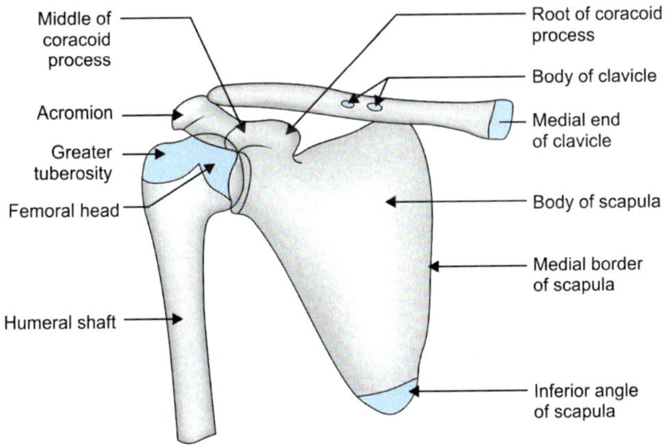


**Fig. 12.9:** Shoulder joint

**Table 12.8:** Wrist and hand

| **Bones** | **Ossification** | |
|---|---|---|
| Capitate | 4 months | |
| Hamate | 4 months | |
| Triquetral | 3 years | |

*Contd...*

*Contd...*

| | | |
|---|---|---|
| Lunate | 4–5 years | |
| Trapezium | 6 years | |
| Trapezoid | 6 years | |
| Capitate | 6 years | |
| Scaphoid | 6 years | |
| Pisiform | 11 years | |
| Metacarpals | 10th week of fetal life | |
| Proximal phalanges | 11th week of fetal life | |
| Middle phalanges | 12th week of fetal life | |
| Distal phalanges | 9th week of fetal life | |
| Middle phalanx of 5th digit | 14th week of fetal life | |
| **Epiphysis** | **Appearance** | **Fusion** |
| Lower end of radius | 1–2 years | 20th year |
| Lower end of ulna | 5–8 years | 20th year |
| Metacarpal heads | 2.5 years | 20th year |
| Base of proximal phalanges | 2.5 years | 20th year |
| Base of middle phalanges | 3 years | 18–20 years |
| Base of distal phalanges | 3 years | 18–20 years |
| Base of 1st metacarpal | 2.5 years | 20th year |

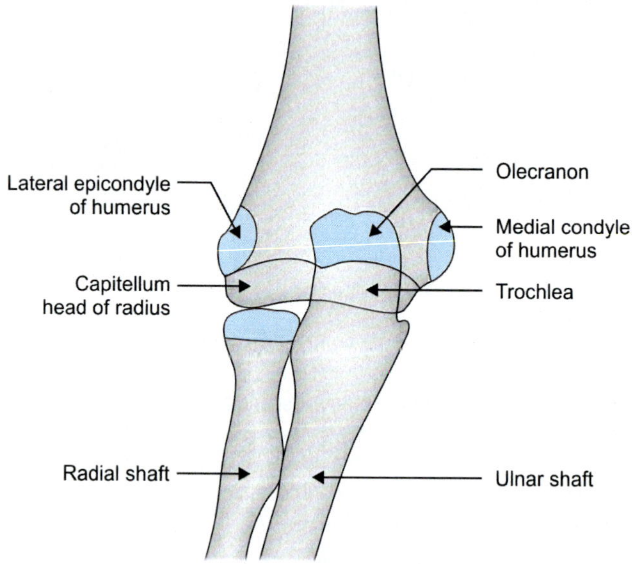


**Fig. 12.10:** Elbow joint

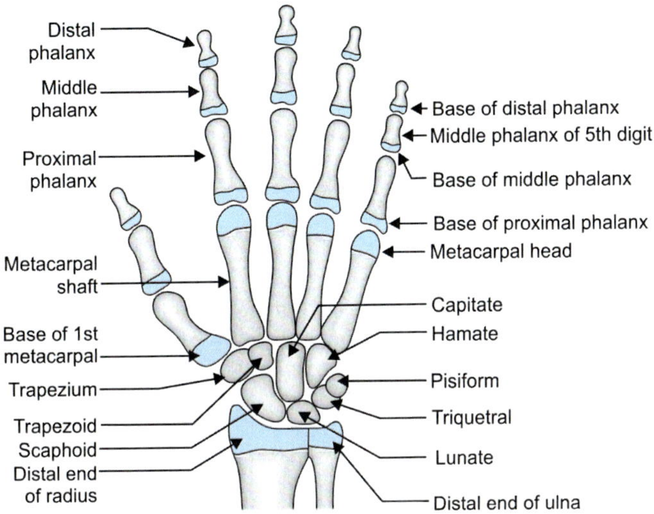


Fig. 12.11: Wrist and hand

Table 12.9: Hip joint

| Bones | Ossification | |
|---|---|---|
| Proximal femoral shaft | 7th week of fetal life | |
| **Epiphysis** | **Appearance** | **Fusion** |
| Femoral head | 1 year | 18–20 years |
| Greater trochanter | 3–5 years | 18–20 years |
| Lesser trochanter | 8–14 years | 18–20 years |

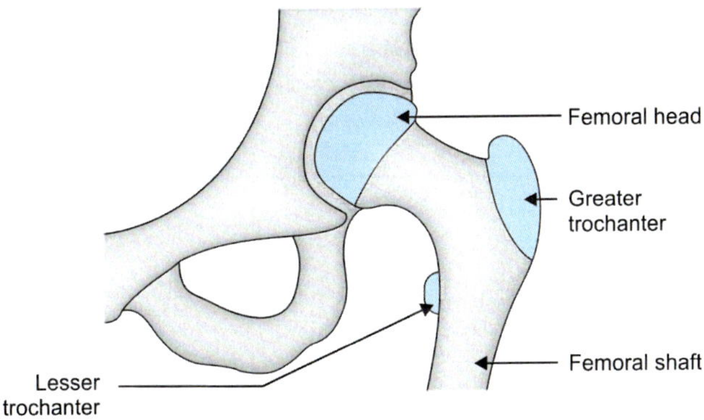


Fig. 12.12: Hip joint

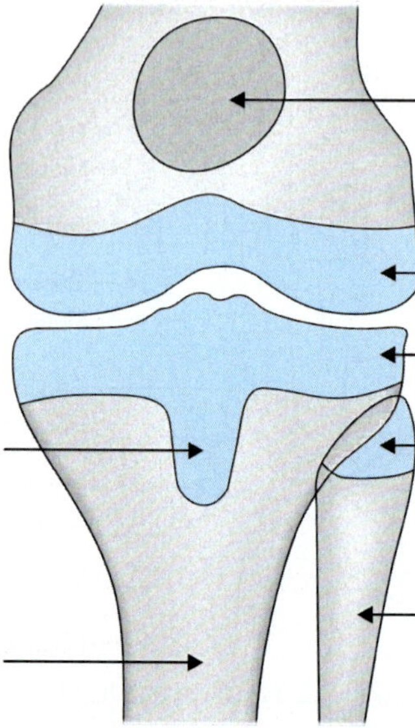


**Fig. 12.13:** Knee joint

**Table 12.10:** Knee joint

| Bones | Ossification | |
|---|---|---|
| Tibial shaft | 7th week of fetal life | |
| Fibular shaft | 8th week of fetal life | |
| Patella | 5 years | |
| **Epiphysis** | **Appearance** | **Fusion** |
| Proximal tibia | At birth | 20th year |
| Tibial tubercle | 5–10 years | 20th year |
| Proximal fibular | 4th year | 25th year |
| Distal femur | At birth | 20th year |

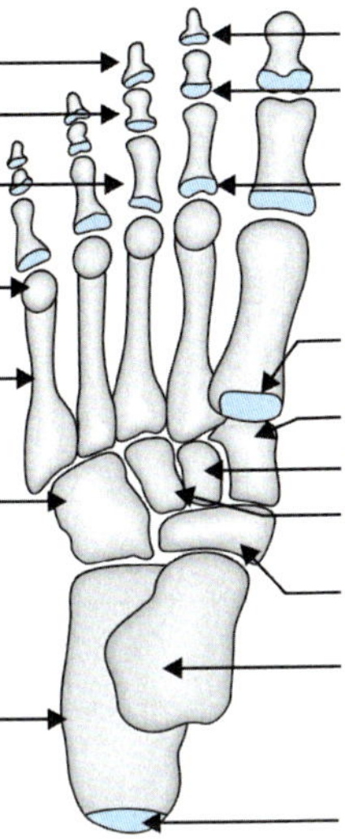


**Fig. 12.14:** Foot and ankle

**Table 12.11:** Foot and ankle

| Bones | Ossification | |
|---|---|---|
| Calcaneus | 6th month of fetal life | |
| Talus | 6th month of fetal life | |
| Navicular | 3-4 years | |
| Cuboid | At birth | |
| Lateral cuneiform | 1 year | |
| Middle cuneiform | 3 years | |
| Medial cuneiform | 3 years | |
| Metatarsal shafts | 8th-9th week of fetal life | |
| Phalangeal shafts | 10th week of fetal life | |
| **Epiphysis** | **Appearance** | **Fusion** |
| Metatarsals | 3 years | 17–20 years |
| Proximal phalangeal base | 3 years | 17–20 years |
| Middle phalangeal base | 3 years | 17–20 years |
| Distal phalangeal base | 5 years | 17–20 years |
| Posterior calcaneal | 5 years | At puberty |

# 13 CHAPTER

# PCPNDT Act

Chapter Outline

- Pre-Birth Sex Selection
- Search and Seize

## PRE-BIRTH SEX SELECTION

Pre-birth Sex selective abortion is the elimination of the female fetus in the womb itself. However, prior to the elimination, the sex of the fetus is determined by amniocentesis or chorion villus biopsy but now by the most popular technique ultrasonography. Once the sex of the fetus is determined as female, it is aborted.

Sonography uses inaudible sound waves to get a visual image of the fetus on a monitor and is normally employed to determine the fetal position or abnormalities, the technique can be used to determine sex if external genitalia of a male fetus is seen. This is possible around 16 weeks of gestation and depends on the position of the fetus in the womb.

Pre-birth Sex selective abortion has brought about abandoning of moral responsibility of few doctors, radiologists, sonologists and geneticists who got involved in discriminatory social practice of son-preference and daughter-aversion. But each time they made profit there was loss of a girl child. When a girl is eliminated an entire generation is wiped out.

Thus the medical community, which has the potential to play a major role in eradicating sex selection, has instead contributed to its prevalence. With these unethical practices multiplying, the medical profession has been under severe pressure to respond to the situation.

To prevent Sex Selection for female feticide Pre-natal Diagnostic Techniques (PNDT) Act 1994 was enacted by parliament and suitably amended Rules have came into effect in 2003 as Pre-conception and Pre-natal Diagnostic Techniques (PCPNDT).

Several bodies representing the medical fraternity immediately took up the issue making the fight against this practice as a part of their agenda.

The PCPNDT law is a prohibitory and regulatory statute; it seeks to put in place a mechanism which prohibits sex selection while preventing the misuse and over-use of the pre-natal diagnostic techniques. The Act permits and regulates the use of such techniques for the purpose of detection of specific genetic abnormalities for the larger benefit of mankind.

By PCPNDT Act it is mandatories for all Genetic Counseling Centers, Genetic Laboratory or Ultrasound Clinics or Imaging Center, whether the body is government, private, voluntary, or contractual to be registered with Appropriate Authority (AA).

Every application has to be accompanied with an affidavit containing an undertaking that is - shall not conduct any test or procedure, by whatever name, for selection of sex before or after conception or for detection of sex of fetus except for specific genetic abnormalities, nor shall the sex of fetus be disclosed to any body.

If any person acts contrary to the Act will be liable to be punished with imprisonment which may extend to 3 years; and fine which may extend to ₹ 10,000/-.

That the said advertisement is in clear violation of different provisions of the PNDT Act which have been reproduced herein below: Prohibition of advertisement relating to pre-natal determination of sex and punishment for contravention. No person, organization, Genetic Counseling Center, Genetic Laboratory or Genetic Clinic, including clinic, laboratory or center having ultrasound machine or imaging machine or scanner or any other technology capable of undertaking determination of sex of fetus or sex selection shall issue, publish, distribute, communicate or cause to be issued, published, distributed or communicated any advertisement, in any form, including internet, regarding facilities of prenatal determination of sex or sex selection before conception available at such center, laboratory, clinic or at any other place.

These records are required to be maintained for a period of 2 years from the date of completion of counseling, pre-natal diagnostic procedure or prenatal diagnostic test or in the event of any legal proceeding, till the final disposal of the legal proceeding.

## SEARCH AND SEIZE

A search is an integral step in a criminal investigation. Whenever an Appropriate Authority or any other authorized officer has reason to believe that an offence under the Act has been or is being committed, he may search a Genetic Counseling center, a Genetic laboratory or Genetic clinic or any other place which is suspected of conducting prenatal diagnostic techniques.

The scope of the powers of the appropriate authority to search and seize is very wide and it includes the power to:

- Enter freely into the place of search.
- Search at all reasonable times.
- Examine and inspect all documents like: i. Registers, ii. Records including consent forms, referral slips charts, laboratory results, and microscopic pictures, iii. Forms, iv. Books, v. Pamphlets, vi. Advertisements, vii. Material objects like sonographic plates or slides, viii. Equipment like ultrasonography machines, needles, fetoscope, etc.
- Seize and seal any document, record, material object or equipment etc. if there is reason to believe that it may furnish evidence of commission of an offence punishable under the Act. It has been clarified that 'material object' would include records, machines and equipments; and 'seize' and 'seizure' would include 'seal' and 'sealing' respectively.

Under the amended Rules, it has been provided that every Genetic Counseling Center, Genetic Laboratory, Genetic Clinic, Ultrasound Clinic, Imaging Center, nursing home, hospital, institute or any other place where any of the machines or equipments capable of performing any procedure, technique or pre-natal determination of sex or selection of sex before or after conception is used, shall afford all reasonable facilities for inspection of the place, equipment and records to the Appropriate Authority in this behalf for registration of such institutions, by whatever name called, under the Act, or for detection of misuse of such facilities or advertisement therefore, or for selection of sex before or after conception, or for detection/disclosure of sex of fetus or for detection of cases of violation of the provisions of the Act in any other manner.

# 14 CHAPTER

# Syllabus

Chapter Outline

- Syllabus in Radiology for Undergraduates

## SYLLABUS IN RADIOLOGY FOR UNDERGRADUATES

### Bones and Joints

Congenital dislocation of hip, congenital syphilis, achondroplasia, osteogenesis imperfecta.

### *Infection*

Osteomyelitis, tuberculosis of bone and spine.

### *Lesions of Joints*

Septic/tuberculous arthritis, rheumatoid, arthritis, ankylosing spondylitis, osteoarthritis, gout.

### *Bone Tumors*

Ewing's, osteogenic sarcoma, giant cell tumor.

### *Lymphoreticular System and Hemopoietic Disorders*

Thalassemia, sickle cell disease, lymphomas, multiple myeloma, plasmacytoma, hemophilia.

### *Metabolic and Endocrine Disorders of Bone*

Rickets and osteomalacia, scurvy, osteoporosis, acromegaly, and hyperparathyroidism.

### *Skeletal Trauma*

General principles.

### Chest

Methods of examination, normal X-ray chest, bronchopulmonary segments.

### Interpretation of Abnormal Chest X-ray

Silhouette sign, air bronchogram, interstitial shadows, alveolar shadows, honeycomb lung, cavitation, calcification, hilar shadow, mediastinum, pleura.

Bronchography, bronchogenic carcinoma.

Miliary shadows, pulmonary tuberculosis, solitary pulmonary nodule, bronchiectasis, primary complex.

### Cardiovascular System

#### *Normal heart*

Methods of examination, cardiomegaly, pericardial effusion.

#### *Acquired Heart Diseases*

Valvular heart disease, ischemic heart disease.

Congenital heart disease.

Aortic aneurysm, coarctation of the aorta.

### Gastrointestinal Tract and Abdomen

Barium examination of gastrointestinal tract. Acute abdomen.

#### *Esophagus*

Carcinoma, strictures, varices, achalasia, and hiatus hernia.

#### Stomach and Duodenum

Ulcer disease, malignancy.

#### *Intestine*

Intestinal obstruction, volvulus, ulcerative colitis, intussusception, malignancy, Hirschsprung's disease, Koch's abdomen, diverticular disease, polyp's.

### Hepatobiliary System and Pancreas

#### *Liver*

Abscess, hepatoma, cirrhosis, portal hypertension, and splenoportography.

### *Gallbladder*

Calculus disease, malignancy, PTC, ERCP.

### Pancreas

Pancreatitis, malignancy.

## Uroradiology, Obstetrics and Gynecology

### *Method of Examination*

Intravenous urography (IVP)

Calculus disease, PUJ obstruction, PU valves, renal artery stenosis, wilm's tumor, renal cell carcinoma, genitourinary Koch's.

Hysterosalpingography (HSG), intrauterine fetal death, fibroid, ovarian tumors, ultrasonography and transvaginal US.

## Central Nervous System

Raised intracranial tension, intracranial calcification, head injury, cerebrovascular accident, ring enhancing lesions in brain, spinal neoplasms, myelograpy.

### *Miscellaneous*

Radiation hazards, radiation protection.

## Imaging Modalities

### *USG, CT, MRI*

Principles, applications, advantages, limitations, developments.

### *Angiography*

Seldinger technique, conventional angiogram, DSA, carotid, coronary, renal angiograms, aortogram.

### *Contrast Media*

Barium sulfate, water soluble and oily contrast.

### *Interventional Radiology*

Developments, angioplasty, embolization.

### *Mammography*

Principles and applications.

# Index

Page numbers followed by *f* refer to figure and *t* refer to table

## C

S



T

## U



## V



## W



## X